GIACI AND ME

GIACI AND ME

A Mother's Journey of Loving and
Raising an Autistic Child

RITA MICELI

POWNAL STREET PRESS
CHARLOTTETOWN

Giaci and Me: A Mother's Journey of Loving and Raising an Autistic Child. Text copyright © 2024 by Rita T. Miceli.

Pownal Street Press · www.pownalstreetpress.com

All rights reserved. No part of this book may be reproduced, stored in a retrieval system or transmitted, in any form or by any means, without the prior written permission of the author except in the case of brief quotations embodied in reviews.

Requests for permission to make copies of any part of the work should be emailed to permissions at hello@pownalstreetpress.com. Our books may be purchased for promotional, educational, or business use. Please contact your local bookseller or Pownal Street Press at hello@pownalstreetpress.com to purchase.

Cataloguing data available from Library and Archives Canada

ISBN 978-1-998129-00-3 (Paperback) · ISBN 978-1-998129-13-3 (Ebook)

Edited by Mo Duffy Cobb · Designed by Jordan Beaulieu · Author and cover photo by Rita Miceli.

This is a work of creative nonfiction. All the events in this collection are true to the best of the author's memory. It reflects the author's present recollections of experiences over time. Some names and identifying features may have been changed to protect the identity of certain parties. Some events have been compressed, and some dialogue has been recreated. The author in no way represents any company, corporation or brand mentioned herein.

The author has made every attempt to provide information that is accurate and complete in accordance with subjective, personal experience, but this book is not intended as a substitute for professional medical advice. This book is not meant to be used, nor should it be used, to diagnose or treat any medical or psychological condition. Neither the author nor Pownal Street Press are liable for any outcome that may result from a reader's interpretation of the information presented in this memoir.

Pownal Street Press gratefully acknowledges Mi'kma'ki, the ancestral and unceded territory of the Mi'kmaq First Nation on whose land our office is located.

Printed and bound in Canada by Marquis.

28 27 26 25 24 1 2 3 4 5

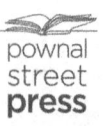

pownal
street
press

To John,

for authenticating our life's journey with love,
integrity, humility, and perseverance,
and to our children for guiding the way.

Contents

PREFACE	9
PART ONE: IN THE BEGINNING	11
ONE: 960 Minutes	12
TWO: I Wanna Dance!	18
THREE: An Italian Connection	23
FOUR: A Home Filled with Little Ones	30
FIVE: His Name Fits	35
SIX: A Fierce Panic	41
SEVEN: "He'll Catch Up, Right?"	46
EIGHT: Why My Son?	53
NINE: A Race Against Time	57
TEN: The Wrestling Game	59
ELEVEN: A True Puzzle	67
TWELVE: Teachable Moments	76
THIRTEEN: Play Date	81
FOURTEEN: Twin Sisters	88
FIFTEEN: "Holy Crap, Lauren!"	95
PART TWO: AT THE THRESHOLD	98
SIXTEEN: ABA Is Evidence-Based Therapy	99
SEVENTEEN: Let's Get to Work	109

EIGHTEEN: "His Hearing Is Fine"   117

NINETEEN: I Need Help!   123

TWENTY: Ambiguous Loss   130

TWENTY-ONE: The "Cut-Off" Age   137

TWENTY-TWO: Fired Up in the Courthouse   143

TWENTY-THREE: Getting a Haircut   149

TWENTY-FOUR: Such Hurtful Words   152

TWENTY-FIVE: The Old-School Mentality   159

TWENTY-SIX: Let Go and Trust God   165

TWENTY-SEVEN: An Italian-Style Field Trip   170

PART THREE: TRANSFORMATION   176

TWENTY-EIGHT: Reaching Out   177

TWENTY-NINE: Two Mothers on a Mission   183

THIRTY: A Mother's Wishful Thinking   191

THIRTY-ONE: A Horrific Night   196

THIRTY-TWO: "What Will Others Think" Syndrome   205

THIRTY-THREE: A Father's Release   220

THIRTY-FOUR: "Normal" Family Activities   229

THIRTY-FIVE: Disney Bliss   241

THIRTY-SIX: Fear of the Future   247

THIRTY-SEVEN: An Unconventional Route   256

THIRTY-EIGHT: A Happy-Go-Lucky Young Man   261

THIRTY-NINE: Two Different Paths   265

FORTY: The Fullness of Life   270

Preface

> One day you will tell your story of how you overcame what you went through, and it will be someone else's survival guide.
>
> —BRENÉ BROWN

Being active and visible in my local autism community, I have often been asked to tell our family's story. Here it is, raw and unfiltered—my honest thoughts and vulnerabilities revealed against the backdrop of my strong Italian upbringing.

This is a story about my son Giaci (pronounced *Judgy*), who during infancy was like every other little boy until we noticed he lacked language and began to demonstrate odd behaviours. By the time he reached the age of two, we received an explanation when Giaci was diagnosed with autism.

Giaci and Me: A Mother's Journey of Loving and Raising an Autistic Child invites the reader into my family's world and shows how we evolved through decades of education, of struggle, and of growth. Be warned! It depicts my stubbornness and desperation in wanting my son to live with me in my world, and not the sound of emptiness that he preferred.

When I began this journey of my son's diagnosis with autism, I felt alone. I would have loved to have heard another mother's story of the peaks and valleys that come with watching a family member with autism grow into adulthood, and how her entire family dealt with it along the way.

But unfortunately, at that time, no such book was available. So I journaled about our process, and it gave me the chance to disclose my innermost feelings about having to contend with autism daily. Even when I was too busy or too exhausted to write out my thoughts, subjects for possible journal entries swirled through my head, and I would make sure to write them down. I've incorporated these passages into this book, which conveys my state of mind as our journey unfolded.

This book is for parents whose children have been diagnosed with autism or any other type of developmental disability; my hope is that reading about my struggles and the lessons I learned may make the path easier for them. As an educator with more than thirty years of experience, I can add a teacher's perspective, especially on the importance of turning every experience into a potential learning opportunity and establishing a foundation of solid expectations and consistency.

Autism doesn't affect just the child; it affects the whole family. For this reason, family, friends and professionals in the field will find this book helpful—an aid to more fully understanding the depths of one family's emotional journey to better serve families with an autistic loved one.

Giaci and Me: A Mother's Journey of Loving and Raising an Autistic Child explores faith, culture and family. It is about trusting ourselves and the people around us. It is about having the courage to persevere and to love wholeheartedly.

Even though my autism journey is unique to me, I am sure you will find guideposts for your own journey. I am honoured to share this story with you.

PART ONE

In the Beginning

ONE

960 Minutes

I sat on the edge of the bed, breastfeeding the twins in a football hold, listening to my son squeal as he ran in circles. The days looped, being both predictable and erratic. The laundry was folded, the meals were cooked, the kitchen was cleaned. Yet in that moment I couldn't remember doing any of it. I was on autopilot; everything I did felt robotic.

I looked at the stacks of boxes. It had been six months since we'd moved into this house. The dining room looked like a storage unit, with no furniture and a mountain of boxes that blocked the window. The walls were bare. I could barely see the labels on the boxes, or had I labelled them? *I could unpack while the twins nap,* I thought, *or it could be an activity for Giaci and Lauren—they could help some.* But that level of management, supervision and organization was too much work. If I opened the boxes, where would I put the items?

After burping the twins, I placed them on the changing mat. They looked "normal," just as their three-year-old sister, Lauren, had. But then again, so had my son Giaci at that age. The diaper changes for three took up most of the day—a constant rotation of clean, dirty, dirty, clean. After changing their diapers, I put the twins in their cribs for naps while Lauren tried to engage her two-year-old brother. She sat on the kitchen floor, piling up the pots and pans as high as she could reach so her brother could knock them down. But he didn't. It was as though I lived in a mini daycare with no support staff.

The next morning, the cycle was repeated. John got up at the same time, dressed in a suit and tie and went to his municipal government office job. He kissed my forehead and left. As soon as he left, I began counting down the minutes until he returned.

John was gone 720 minutes each day. After the office, he'd come home for dinner, change into old sweatpants and steel-toed boots, and then leave to go to his second job of construction work for another 240 minutes. A total of 960 long minutes.

After John left one morning, I covered my head with the bedsheets. I lay frozen and quietly for a few more minutes, absorbing the silence of the bedded cave. I relished the moments before all four of my little ones were fully awake. But always before too long, the twins would stir, and soon their cries would fill the room again.

Once I was up, I pumped breastmilk with one hand and vacuumed with the other as I pushed toys into a corner. While putting away the twins' clothes, I found melted butter in the closet, all over their little shoes. *This is too much.* I didn't remember doing this. I closed the closet door and, pretending I didn't see it, went to check on the kids. I'd clean it up later.

Lauren and Giaci were still snuggling together on their queen-sized bed in their *Sesame Street*-themed bedroom. We kept them together in one bigger bed so Lauren could comfort her brother if he woke up in the middle of the night. This helped him sleep more soundly—or so we hoped. No matter how tired Lauren may have been, she kept one arm wrapped around him, and he didn't wander off in the night.

When they awoke, I greeted them individually. "Good morning, Giaci! Good morning, Lauren!" I hoped I'd get a response from both, but Giaci didn't say anything.

"Morning, Mommy!" Ever chipper in the morning, Lauren snapped up as soon as she saw me. Lauren was a motormouth, rambling on and on about her Barbies and their outfits. Giaci, though energetic throughout the day, took his time in the morning. He wiped his sleepy green eyes and lay there smiling as I walked over to get him out of his heavy diaper and into clean clothes. His tousled golden-brown hair stood upright on one side of his head, and he flapped his hands up and down. Within no time, Giaci was at his highest energy level, running donuts on the carpet in his bedroom, around the scattered Polly Pocket toys. The trash can beside the change table was full, and the stench of dirty diapers hung in the air—and it clung to me.

The wall clock caught my eye. Eight hundred more minutes until John would be home.

Nights consisted of feedings and Giaci bouncing around and squealing. Some nights I barely slept for an hour. When I needed a shower to wake me up for the day, I had a program. I had to bring all my children into the bathroom with me, which left little privacy for an emotional release.

I locked the door to secure their safety and made sure that the twins were in their car seats, and that Giaci and Lauren had enough toys to entertain them.

"Lauren, honey, please be a big girl for Mommy and watch over your little brother and sisters while I take a quick shower. I know how much you love them, and I know you will do a good job," I said as I slipped behind the curtain.

I needed to rely on my three-and-a-half-year-old's nurturing instincts for help as it was the only way to get five minutes to myself. But even then, showering wasn't what it once had been. The warm steam felt nice against my skin, but the comfort was constantly interrupted as I peeked around the shower curtain every thirty seconds, making sure that everyone was still occupied and locked in the bathroom with me. Giaci didn't understand danger and was always ready to dart off. Lauren blocked his exit and gave him a talking to. I hurried to finish up.

Giaci jumped and flapped his hands, squeaking with a high-pitched voice. "No Giaci, sit down, Mommy needs a shower, so stop it."

He continued.

I had known motherhood would be hard, but I hadn't imagined it would be this hard.

In the shower, the fear and confusion I hid inside seeped out through my pores. I thought about every moment of anger. I resented the disorder that lurked within my child and drained me of the energy I needed to care for all my babies. I could hear Lauren trying to engage her brother with the Lego blocks. She begged him to knock them down. "Look Giaci, look." But he didn't respond. Nothing.

It did this to our family, to me. *Autism* did this.

While in the shower, I said the word out loud for the first time, even though it was still just a whisper. *Autism.* Three months before the twins were born, Giaci had been given this diagnosis, and I had barely begun to process it. With his diagnosis came many unknowns, and it was tearing me apart inside. *Would he ever be able to communicate? Would he ever be able to have friends? How will he live?* I had four wonderful children, but this autism diagnosis made me feel like a failure as a mother. I wasn't prepared for it. Processing it left me anxious, confused and scatterbrained. I wondered, *Is anyone ever prepared for an autism diagnosis?* The fear of an unknown future scared me. My husband was hardworking and devoted, yet in our own unique ways, I felt as though we were both going through the motions of not breaking down. We didn't speak of it because it hurt so much. The fear of the unknown was evident in our eyes. When I would look at him and he at me, we would tear up and become incommunicative. We functioned in silence.

"The cow says 'moo!'" came from Giaci's toy on the other side of the shower curtain.

Again and again he pulled the lever of his toy, which kept repeating "The cow says 'moo!'" and "The cow says 'moo!'" and "The cow says—" I couldn't take it anymore. The reruns of the day were debilitating. I was stuck on a nursery-school hamster wheel, spinning, running in one spot.

My mind raced, and all I could think about was that there were around 630 minutes to go. *Ten and a half hours until John comes home.*

I needed to tell John how I was feeling. Not talking about our son's diagnosis made it that much harder to digest. I felt powerless against autism, a foe that was becoming stronger every day. Giaci was being pulled deeper into his own world, content with little human interaction and continual repetitive behaviours. To me, autism and my beautiful little boy were two separate entities. At least I wished they were. I wanted to separate them. In my eyes, my son was innocent, adorable and sweet. Autism was heartless and cruel.

I stayed in the shower a bit longer than usual, blocking out the toddler energy on the other side of the curtain. I shut the water off. I didn't even have the will to be present in my kids' joy, not when we had an unknown entity among us, creeping beneath the surface. It was as if a thief had come in the night and robbed my perfect boy of his soul, leaving me just the outer shell. On the outside, Giaci looked like every other child. But it seemed as if on the inside, parts of him were missing, and I longed to unlock the doors that separated us.

As I dressed behind the curtain, I began to shake with insurmountable anger as I put on yoga pants yet again. *I shouldn't have let this happen,* I thought. I felt that, as his mother, I should have fought this disorder away. But I hadn't. I had been blindsided. Defenceless.

Autism had stolen all the potential of my child's normal life and had left us with a blank slate.

I opened the shower curtain. "Thank you, Lauren, for watching Giaci and your sisters."

"You're welcome, Mommy," she said, smiling, pleased as I forced a grin to acknowledge my appreciation.

Days passed. Weeks passed. All continued like the one before. And still, my son did not speak.

After I put the kids to bed, life stood still. I sat down on the couch, waiting in silence for some adult conversation. *Ninety more minutes, then John will be home.* Silence. Waiting. *John will be home in an hour and a half.*

When the front door opened, I jumped up eagerly to tell John all about our waking hours, the day's discoveries, Lauren's courage, Giaci's *moo*. But at the end of his own long day, John didn't have much left for connection. He would plop down his tool belt and take off his work boots. A quick bite and he would walk with heavy steps toward the bedroom, his eyes half open. I followed close behind him.

He would crash almost immediately upon getting into bed, and I was left lying there.

Zero minutes.

John was home, but I still felt so alone.

TWO

I Wanna Dance!

My life hadn't always been so overwhelming, and I hadn't always felt so alone. When I was a teenager, I was very sheltered. I had a sweet, naive look when I smiled, and I wasn't allowed to venture out alone. In the 1980s, when I was growing up and coming of age, everyday life was quite different from the way it is today.

My family lived in the core of Little Italy, an overpopulated, predominantly Italian immigrant neighbourhood in Windsor, Ontario. The aroma of fresh tomato sauce on the stove was constant. On the clothesline, bedsheets snapped in the wind and smelled like sunshine. Homes were situated close to each other, almost on top of each other. Without propping our windows open, even with the television on, we could hear our Italian-speaking neighbours' conversations.

You gotta eat. Mangia.

Go help your mother. Aiuta la mamma.

Don't hit your sister. Lascia stare la tua sorella.

My dad defined my understanding of the word *protector*. He was my umbrella in the rain, always sparing me from any kind of pain of being hurt physically or emotionally. But I just wanted to grow up.

It was the spring of 1986, and I wanted to go to a high school dance, but my parents refused. They were overprotective, strict Italian immigrants who felt the need to safeguard me from the chaotic world around me. It was an Old World mentality. Behind my father's unwillingness to let me go to the school dance was the unasked question: *What would the neighbours think if young Rita were allowed to go out dancing?* As if I would be regarded as a floozy for associating with my peers, even under the watchful eye of school officials. I was from a respectable family, and I didn't dare bring shame to it.

"Daddy, *please* let me go to the dance, *please!*" I asked persistently. "I'll do the laundry, I'll do extra homework, I'll do anything!" I pleaded with my hands gripped together.

"Why you wanna go there?" he asked, not understanding the desire I had to enjoy some time with my friends. I knew it was because he didn't like the fact that boys would be there, without his watchful eyes keeping them away from me. It didn't seem like he was going to let me go. But much to my surprise, after days of pestering my dad about it, he finally agreed.

The night of the dance was a breezy one. I donned my high-waisted, skinny-fit whitewashed jeans and a bright pink polyester shirt with thick shoulder pads, ready to fit in with the '80s crowd. My stomach tensed with anticipation as I got into the passenger seat of my dad's 1968 emerald-green Ford Fairlane. I reached into the front pocket of my pants to make sure I had cash, the money I earned from my paper route.

Don't change your mind. Don't change your mind, I prayed. The typical Italian immigrant parenting style was very guarded. I wasn't allowed to venture off into anything out of the ordinary and always had to stay close to home and family. Schoolwork, housework, and family time were on the itinerary every day. But just this once I wanted to add a school dance to the schedule, and it was happening!

I prayed with my eyes closed the entire ride there. I only opened them when we stopped and I found myself in front of my school. I fumbled out of the door with a rushed "Bye, Daddy!" as I slammed the door shut behind me.

I stutter-stepped my way to the school's cement steps. Dad was still there in his car, watching and waiting. My heart sped up. He glared at everyone in sight, as if he were the head of my security team. I bit my lip, hoping he wouldn't change his mind at the last minute. Step by step, I inched closer to freedom. I realized that I was exchanging the safe haven of home and family for a new and exciting experience. A wave of anxiety swept over me.

I walked into the gymnasium with a cautious smile. *Am I really at the dance?* After glancing at the face of Queen Elizabeth II on the crumpled dollar bill I'd pulled out of my pocket, I paid the entrance fee to my classmate who was sitting at the admission table. Having passed that hurdle, I pumped my fist in the air in celebration and then relaxed as my inner voice cheered, *Woo-hoo! I made it! Let's dance!*

My tensed stomach quickly turned into butterflies dancing. Suddenly, through the blaring '80s dance music, I heard my pulse in my ears. Young MC's "Bust a Move," Whitney Houston's "I Wanna Dance with Somebody," and Newcleus's breakdance staple "Jam on It" were a few of the welcoming numbers. All dance-goers had to take their shoes off at the door, so as not to scratch the shiny wooden gym floor. To the left of the gymnasium doors was a sea of Converse and Adidas running shoes and women's flats, all smelling like sweaty feet. No one pinched their nose. Everyone ignored it.

A multitude of teenagers in white sweat socks walked around, chattering, laughing, and dancing to the top hits of the '80s. It was just as I had envisioned it. I was ready to show off my dance moves. With my teased hair, which was easily the height of a vertical pencil and sprayed with layers of Aqua Net hairspray, I searched for my girlfriends. They weren't too difficult to find, since they too had curly, dark brown, backcombed hair with thick bangs.

"Hey, guys!" I yelled over the loud music. "Hey!"

They waved and approached me.

"You guys look great."

"You too," they answered in unison.

"I can't believe I'm here," I said.

"Let's go dance."

We grabbed each other's hands and walked farther into the cloud of music. Giggling and carefree, we hit the dance floor with popular breakdance moves like the wave and the windmill. Dancing liberated my nerves and excitement.

As I danced, I sensed eyes on me. Someone was watching me from the bleachers that rose along the outer perimeter of the gym. One broad-shouldered teenaged boy, sitting with his posse of guy friends, was ogling me. His hair was cut short on the front and sides but left long at the back—a perfect mullet. He had a peach-fuzz moustache with a few pimples spotted across his oily face, and he wore a high school football city championship leather jacket paired with baggy-fit stone-washed jeans.

I pointed him out to my friends, and my girlfriend Lu recognized him. They had attended the same elementary school.

"John is looking at you!" she said with a smirk.

I turned to look fully. John's eyes met mine. We were drawn to each other by a magnetic force.

He didn't join us at first, but when a slow song came on, he walked over and gently tapped me on the shoulder.

"Rita, right?" he said, barely audible over the music.

"Yes," I answered as I turned to face him.

He gestured toward the dance floor.

My heart did somersaults, and I moved in his direction like Pinocchio, with stiff wooden legs.

Immediately there was a natural affinity between us. He smelled delicious, doused in Drakkar Noir cologne by Guy Laroche and chewing strawberry-flavoured Hubba Bubba bubble gum.

We couldn't talk much because the music was ear-shatteringly loud.

We just swayed side to side, barely touching, barely moving to Foreigner's "I Want to Know What Love Is." After the song ended, we went our separate ways, back to our respective circles of friends.

My girlfriends were giddy, hugging me as if I had accomplished something spectacular. I blushed, but my internal voice kept saying, *Keep cool, girl, keep cool.* I struggled to keep cool, though, because my naive inner thoughts were focused on one thing: *He's the one.*

Before I knew it, it was time for my father to pick me up. I hurried to the door and raced down the steps, just like Cinderella fleeing the ball. But instead of fearing my gown and carriage would melt away when the clock struck twelve, my concern was Dad getting out of the car or doing anything to embarrass me in front of my friends.

I quickly jumped into the car.

"Hi, Daddy."

"Hi, you have a good time?" he asked, straight-faced.

"Yeah, it was OK." I downplayed it. I didn't dare tell him I had a blast and that I danced with a boy. He may have regretted letting me go.

I'd gone to the dance just to have a good time, but I left knowing I'd met the love of my life.

John was the one.

THREE

An Italian Connection

At the beginning of the next school year, in grade twelve, John and I started seeing each other. Like our first dance, our courtship was slow and steady. We talked mainly at school or at home on our telephones—landlines, of course. I wasn't allowed to date, so our relationship was chaste. John completely understood; he had been raised with the same old-school rules. In a traditional Italian family, daughters must remain safely under the protective eyes of their parents, while sons are allowed to venture out.

John came over to my house often. That was how our teenage courtship went: under the watchful eyes of my parents.

At the local Italian supermarket, Mom had heard that John was a good boy; the fact that he was Italian helped, too.

John became a regular visitor, mostly sitting on the couch with Dad, speaking in Italian about life in Italy versus life in Canada. My job was to serve them coffee and desserts. The gender roles were clear in our household, and because John understood, no explanation was needed. I had occasional moments of jealousy that I wasn't treated the way my brothers were, but I didn't make a fuss. It made our courtship easier, and that's how it had to be.

"Gianni, you wanna coffee?" Mom would call out from the kitchen when John arrived.

"Yes, thank you!" John answered politely.

The languages bounced back and forth seamlessly: sometimes Italian and other times English.

One day, while mom poured the espresso, I listened to John and Dad talk about the economic downfall of Italy. After the Second World War, it had been especially difficult to live in Italy. There was no work to be found, so no one could feed their families, let alone pay for modern necessities such as indoor plumbing, telephones, refrigeration, and central heating for the cold winters.

So, my family (and John's) emigrated to Canada in search of a better life—a life of opportunities. But both our families were proud of their heritage and kept the culture alive in Canada through the way they raised their children.

As I approached them with the cannoli, Dad was telling John about the hardships he had endured in Partinico, Palermo.

"I worked with the *camio* making the streets in the *paese!*" He described truck driving, poor transportation, and infrastructure in his hometown. He lived not knowing when his next meal would be.

"*La fame,*" he said. *Hunger.* He drew his hand in a repetitive circle over his stomach and stretched out the words to emphasize the magnitude of the hunger he'd experienced.

John listened intently, evaluating every word. He knew how to show respect to his elders, and it made me love him that much more. With European parents, you couldn't wait until they stopped talking to get a word in because that might never happen—you had to find the slightest lull and then jump in with your own story. John knew when to take his opportunity, and he began telling Dad stories about his own father's hard work as a farmer in the fields of Montallegro, Agrigento.

"They never wasted an ounce of food," John said. "If the bread had ants on it, they would blow them off and still eat the bread!"

Dad nodded. "Ya, of course! Becausa you could not waste anything."

I retreated to the kitchen and watched their bond grow. It was clear to Dad that John had it in his blood to cope and to persevere, and that was good enough for his princess.

***

For the next several years, our days were busy. John and I finished high school and stayed together through university.

I pursued an undergraduate degree in French language studies, and John a business degree. Our parents taught us not to fear hard work, but rather to welcome it. To them, working hard meant seven days a week and no time for leisure activities. As a result, John and I were never the type to party every weekend.

Being given the opportunity for a higher education was a privilege that previous generations never had. Dad often said that without an education, our options were limited and that he didn't want us to have a hard life like he did. He wanted us to use our minds, not our hands.

Maintaining our parents' ethic of "all work and no play" was taxing, but it was all we knew. This did not cause generational conflicts; there was joy and fulfillment with our every success, which only confirmed to our parents that they had made the right choice in leaving their homeland.

Both our mothers were frugal, stay-at-home moms, constantly cooking and cleaning. Italian homes are always pristine in case an unexpected visitor decides to pop in, and our mothers ensured that this manicured look was maintained. Child rearing was also mainly our mothers' responsibility, as was grocery shopping, and they both knew how to stretch a penny. They never paid full price for anything. If it was on sale, then it was for dinner. They both cut stacks of coupons every week, and there were always reminders that every penny was hard-earned.

Like our dads, our moms had not been given the opportunity to go to school. John's mom married at eighteen and then she and her new husband immediately started their family. Now she had her hands full with six children: Dino, John, Martino, Vince, Josie and Rosangela. My mother had the three of us, and she would also take on sewing jobs at home to help with the family finances, making draperies or whatever else anyone would pay her to make. When I was a child, she was forever sewing, and sometimes even staying up until the dawn.

Mom kept her sewing machine in a corner of our basement, which was damp and musty, with cement blocks for walls. The ceiling wood studs were exposed. Next to her Singer sewing machine was a homemade table. She had glued a sheet of Formica, a laminate material, to a piece of wood and screwed table legs to it. This was where she cut bolts of fabric. My most vivid memory of her sewing was the red velvet drapes she made for practically every Italian family in the community. The fabric was thick and difficult to work with, but she would get the job done, despite her sore, stiff hands. The fibres stuck to our clothes for months, and we had red velvet remnants all over the house. Her customers were always pleased with her skills and they spread the word, which kept the work coming.

When I was a child, she made my outfits, too. My favourite was a green jumpsuit, tailored to fit me perfectly. After I watched her put the fabric pieces together one step at a time, I was incredibly proud to wear it! Knowing that my mom had stitched it especially for me made it a true one-of-a-kind garment.

As I grew up, she also worked on fancy ballgowns, custom fit. My yellow beaded prom dress was pageant worthy. It had a sweetheart neckline and a bodice that fit me like a silk glove. The sleeves were big and round and covered with pale yellow pearls and sequins. Each bead was sewn individually, stitch by stitch. There was soft, flowery lace on the sleeves and from my waist down to the ground. After I begged, Mom finally agreed to give me a high slit, which revealed perhaps a little too much of my well-tanned leg. To find some middle ground, she sewed a few strands of pearls that dangled there, covering my thigh a little bit more. This dress made me feel like a real princess, and the fact that my mom created it made it that much more special.

In the evenings, after she had sewn for most of the day, Mom cooked and cleaned for our family. She ran around the kitchen, preparing rich Italian meals that she served as soon as Dad got home from the barbershop. I admired her tenacity. I too wanted to be a mother someday, but I also wanted more. Becoming a professional would bring greater financial freedom.

John knew that, too. When I told him that I wanted to further my education and work on a master's degree in education, he took my hand, looked at me with his big eyes, and said, "Rita, my love, I'm proud of you and will stand by you with whatever makes you happy." He brushed my hair aside with his wide hand and winked at me, adding, "We gonna make it."

It was something Dad had often said to encourage me, and John had adopted it. He always knew just what to say to bring air back into my lungs. He knew that I wouldn't be happy as a housewife. I wanted to have it all: career and children, wealth and happiness.

As young people, John and I both charged hard in pursuit of our dreams. After we finished our schooling, John was hired by the municipal government. Even though we were different from our parents, John still felt the need to provide for our future family-to-be and continued to climb in his career.

For me, a degree in education meant making a difference in students' lives. When I was around young children, I felt uplifted. They fascinated me as their young personalities emerged. I was enthralled by their growth. I knew I wanted to be the kind of teacher I would want for my own kids one day.

These professional commitments were the bricks and mortar of the lives we were building. Our financial decisions were based on the philosophy of short-term pain for long-term gain. It was all part of our goal for financial independence, and soon we were well on our way.

* * *

One day in early November of 1991, John asked Dad for my hand in marriage. Of course, Dad gave his blessing, and then John proposed. We were twenty-one years old.

It was custom that we continue down the traditional path with approval from an old-school Italian community. We got to work planning the wedding. As soon as the buzz of our post-secondary graduation wore off, the fierce intensity of wedding festivities was all anyone in our family could talk about. I was the only daughter, sandwiched between two boys—one older brother, Anthony, and one younger brother, David.

By now, John and I were used to juggling multiple responsibilities and projects, and this was no different. In addition to wedding planning, my teaching position, and John's municipal job, we were also building a cozy new home for ourselves. It was a busy time, and we were financially strapped—but as always, we both channelled our focus into accomplishing our every objective.

All the months of spreading ourselves thin finally paid off on our summer wedding day. Of course, it was a big, fat Italian wedding!

John and I were proud of our Italian heritage, and we included many Italian traditions in the wedding. It was 1993, the era of massive hair, and I topped my big hair with a sizable tiara fastened to a long, beaded, white lace bridal veil. My mom stitched every pearl and sequins by hand to my dress and eighteen-foot train. In the Roman Catholic religion, a white veil symbolizes modesty and obedience. We were married in the Italian church, where we paid tribute to the Virgin Mary by placing a bouquet of flowers at the feet of her statue. We also gave out *bonboniere*, the Italian word for "wedding favours." This is a gift given to wedding guests to thank them for attending the wedding. It includes *confetti*—sugar-coated almonds—five for good luck. It was tradition. The almond symbolizes the bittersweetness of marriage and the beginning of a new life.

We couldn't wait to start our life together as husband and wife.

As we said our vows, I could see our happily-ever-after unfolding. I knew in my heart that no matter what life threw our way, we'd solve it together. We had everything we could possibly need because we had each other.

And then we said, "I do."

FOUR

A Home Filled with Little Ones

With my career underway, and with our newly built two-bedroom townhouse complete, we were settling into our new life as a married couple. I was ready for the next step.

One day, as I stood at the counter cutting ripe cantaloupe into half-moons, I felt the words rise out of me:

"I don't want to wait to have children!"

John got up from the table. With his calloused hands, he reached for a slice of cantaloupe as he chewed on my words. He paused as he always did when he was thinking. He turned his eyes toward the ceiling as if he were processing an equation in his head.

Minutes went by, and he still hadn't responded. So, I dramatically filled the silence myself. "I'm afraid I'll have a hard time getting pregnant," I confessed. I hadn't realized how long I'd been holding that in or how heavy it had felt. What if I couldn't have kids? What if I was like my mother, who had a hard time conceiving?

My parents had tried to have children for years and then lost a child due to a ruptured ectopic pregnancy. One of my mother's fallopian tubes had to be removed, leaving her with only one viable side of her reproductive system. Not only had my mother been near death, but her chances of getting pregnant were cut in half.

As older parents who thought their chances of ever having children were slim, they were overjoyed to eventually have three children. They simply never stopped trying or praying. My parents believed that if you prayed hard enough, anything could happen.

This was why we couldn't wait.

The more John considered my words, the more his face revealed his excitement about being a father. He kissed my forehead, and then he leaned back, cocked his head to the side, and winked.

"I think we should start right away," he said.

I responded with an amorous grin. "How's tonight?"

We both laughed and John confirmed, "Food first, of course."

We both wanted kids: I wanted six, and John wanted four. I could imagine them already. Little John running around passing a football back and forth with his dad. Me teaching the girls how to play the piano, beaming as I listened to them perform at recitals. Heavenly thoughts of a home filled with little ones warmed my heart. I couldn't wait to become proud parents, shaping and moulding our children into caring and decent people. It was a dream we could not wait to realize.

As outlandish as my desire for six children probably sounded, John always approached everything with an open mind.

"All right, Ri."

When a month of trying to conceive passed and nothing happened, panic pinched my thoughts. The idea of not being able to have children weighed heavily on me. Because I wanted to be a mother so badly, not being able to conceive would have pulverized my womanhood.

But in John's eyes, I was being overly dramatic. "Relax, Rita. It will happen. The more you worry, the worse it is," he said.

Of course, he was right. In our second month of trying, I became pregnant with our first child.

* * *

With each passing month, my worry eased. I knew this life inside me was meant for us. I felt strong and healthy throughout my pregnancy and continued to teach while experiencing the daily changes in my body.

John was ecstatic every day. He would constantly place his hand on my belly, overjoyed by the movement of his first child.

"Did you feel that kick, honey?" I asked one night, pulling his hand to my belly.

His eyes sparkled as he moved his head toward it. His ear hovered over our unborn child. "I wonder if it's a girl or a boy."

"It doesn't matter as long as he or she is healthy. We'll love them no matter what," I said, knowing this child would complete our home. I was already settling into a maternal role, while John concentrated on his role of primary breadwinner. He had just finished building us another home.

* * *

I went into labour on Tuesday morning, May 3, 1994. We both felt nervous and fearful of the unknown, yet ready to meet this new person we had created.

John grabbed my overnight bag, and we picked up Mom on the way. I staggered between breaths. My contractions were about three minutes apart. It was a piercing pain in my abdomen. I was afraid. *Will this pain get worse? How bad will it get? Can I handle it? How is my unborn child?* My body trembled; labour was frightening.

Trying to maintain an outer display of calmness, John picked up my bag. Despite his best efforts, though, I saw his upper lip twitching. It was clear to me that he was both nervous and excited. We looked at each other for a moment; we knew we were ready for this leap.

As soon as we arrived at the hospital, the nurses checked all my vitals and the baby's heart rate.

One nurse helped me into a wheelchair. "Your chauffeur awaits," she giggled, leading us to the labour and delivery floor.

The nurse got me settled on the bed in a cozy birthing room. It had warm lighting, sky-blue walls, a sink in one corner, and an armchair in another. John sat in a grey stackable chair beside me, his eyes fixed on my every move. Mom stood at the foot of the bed, fastened to the purse in front of her. Her tense body and stiff expression showed her nervousness. I could focus on the two of them only for a moment before my back pain increased and a sharp pelvic ache arose, which pushed me to groan.

As soon as John sat up in his chair, I knew "Coach John" had appeared. He talked me through my plays as he had his football team when he was the captain encouraging his teammates:

"Breathe, honey, breathe. Inhale through your nose. Hold it. Exhale through your mouth. Great job, Rita!" He didn't invade my space as he reminded me of the breathing techniques we had learned in our Lamaze classes.

John continued to coach me through the painful contractions while we waited for the doctor. Beads of sweat appeared on my forehead, and Mom noticed right away. She grabbed a facecloth from the shelf over the corner sink, wet it under the faucet, and handed it to John. He dabbed my forehead. Within minutes, the doctor appeared.

The nurse helped arrange my feet into the stirrups so the doctor could examine me. After the doctor took off his latex gloves, he and the nurse discussed the situation in the far corner of the room. Panic settled in my stomach once again. As my thoughts began to spiral, the doctor returned. He informed us that we were going to have to deliver right away in the operating room.

"The baby is in position, facing head downward. Unfortunately, we'll have to deliver in the operating room as quickly as possible because we've detected meconium. We don't want the baby to aspirate it into the lungs, so it's best we do this now."

Meconium is a thick, sticky substance that can cause problems for a baby's inflating lungs immediately after birth.

I didn't even have time to react. I didn't have any words to say. My hands shook as I grasped the side rails of the hospital bed. Fear mounted in my quivering body and my eyes widened as I focused on John. His presence gave me comfort. The nurses wheeled me into the operating room in the hospital bed I was already on, leaving my mother behind in the hallway.

In the plain, sterile operating room, everyone seemed to move at lightning speed: they had to get the baby out quickly for fear of him or her losing oxygen. The nurse gave John a hospital gown to put on. He shoved his arms into it as he walked behind the moving bed.

Nothing was happening the way I had envisioned; this wasn't the perfect birth story I had wanted. The fear was beyond my control. All I could do was fixate on the yellow stain above me on the off-white ceiling of the cold, sterile operating room.

Everything was prepared in case I needed an emergency Caesarean, but now, thankfully, the nurses prepared for a vaginal birth.

I was zoning in and out, and suddenly, I heard a faint voice say, "Okay, Rita. I'm going to need you to push."

Always an obedient student, I complied and gave it all I had. My heart pounded, almost moving me from my spot, and adrenaline surged through my veins, causing my body to tremble. *Come on*, I thought to my baby. *I need to meet you.*

And with another push, we had a baby girl. I breathed a sigh of relief. When they said she was healthy, I breathed another sigh of relief.

We named her Lauren. *Our* Lauren. She was pale and soft, with the tiniest fingernails I had ever seen. Her eyes were big and steady. She looked up at us, and I could tell she was an old soul. Lauren seemed to have already lived a full life before entering this new, adorable little body. Her sharp gaze told us that she was ready to get to work. She was ready to be part of our team, no matter what.

FIVE

His Name Fits

We were in love and completely and totally overwhelmed (in the best possible way) by joy, responsibility, and selflessness. Lauren was stunning right from the start, with her dark curls and contrasting emerald eyes outlined with velvety eyelashes.

I couldn't think of anything other than her for months. I lived, breathed, and ate her right up. I never truly understood the love of a parent until I became one. It was an all-consuming, unconditional love.

John and I were enchanted by Lauren. As we walked around our third home together, we knew it would never be just the two of us again. We loved every second of it.

Less than a year after having Lauren, I was pregnant with our second baby. It was safe to say that I wasn't worried anymore. Plump and filled with life, I rejoiced over my second go at motherhood. This new member of our family would be just as special; I could feel it.

One day, I looked down at Lauren, who was about one year old, and asked her if she preferred a baby brother or a baby sister.

Lauren had begun to speak early, her first word being *Mama*. As typical as this may have been, discoveries like this were priceless gifts to me. Her personality shone through every day.

"Girl, Mama!" she said, holding up her favourite girl doll, which she played with all the time.

I applauded her efforts with language and scooped her up to carry her to her nursery. We loved spending time there learning and talking while John was at work. The school year had just ended, so I could devote all my attention to Lauren. Seeing her reach all her developmental milestones on time or early made me proud, and it boosted my self-confidence as a mother. She engaged and interacted by pointing to objects or people. This particular day, she was interested in me and my growing belly.

She pointed to my belly and said, "Mama's baby." Then she showed me how she changed her doll's diapers. "I do it, Mama," she said, pinning one strap before the other with perfect patience.

Lauren often acted mature beyond her years. She was incredibly intuitive and soaked up every connection we made for her. She would stay awake as long as she could every day, waiting for her dad to come home. She couldn't wait to tell him what we'd done and learned that day. It was adorable watching John tuck her into bed, and she wouldn't stop talking until she had tired herself out. Sometimes she even fell asleep mid-sentence. John would nod and smile as he took in the earful of chatter that came his way.

Learning from the world around her came easily to Lauren. She absorbed all the lessons life offered. She was a social butterfly, flying from one flower to another and taking in the pollen of conversation. She was also the flower itself, blooming from the sun around her and the water we provided. It was a gift to watch her grow with each passing day.

It made me that much more excited to meet our next child, another version of us—someone who was like me, John, and Lauren, yet with their own spin on things.

When the day came to welcome this new person into our family, I felt much more ready than I had the previous time. There was less fear and more certainty.

As much as Lauren wanted a doll-like girl, it was a boy who came into our lives. I had hit the jackpot: a boy and a girl. It was everything I dreamed of, and a reaffirmation that my life was working out exactly as I had planned it.

Our second child was born on the second of November in 1995, the day after All Saints' Day—a religious holiday commemorating all the saints in the Catholic Church. I was comforted by the meaning of this day and believed the saints were going to grant me another healthy child.

In the labour and delivery room, John's face was bright; he looked the happiest I'd ever seen him. His expression exploded with joy upon seeing his little boy for the first time. He couldn't contain the rush of pride, and a jolly burst of laughter gushed out of him as he repeated after the doctor: "It's a boy."

My mother stood on the sidelines, a fly on the wall. All she said from her corner as they swaddled him was, "The baby came out so *calmo*." She didn't move, not wanting to disrupt the serene scene.

When the nurse passed him to me, his new skin smelled like warm sugared milk, and it was just as smooth and soft to the touch. He filled out the blanket he was wrapped in. He looked just like the Gerber baby. I was in love. I kissed his forehead and promised to protect him forever. I kept my head down and thanked the Lord in prayer. "I know you will give my son the protection he needs," I whispered, adding "Amen."

When I raised my head, I looked at John. "I still think the name fits," I said.

"Me too," he said in a dreamy state, still staring at our boy.

Before the baby's birth, John and I had decided we would follow the Italian tradition of naming our first son after his paternal grandfather, Giacinto. He was a man of few words, but when he spoke, all listened. He was brutally honest and fair, with Herculean strength and a soft heart—much like John.

Lauren was the one to coin his nickname. A few weeks before her brother was born, we had Lauren practise her brother's name.

"Lauren, say Ja-cheen-toe."

"Ja-chee, Ja-chee. That good, Mommy?" she asked, smiling. She shortened it by taking the -nto off.

"That's perfect, honey," I said.

And so his nickname became *Giaci*—pronouncing it *judge-ee*. It sounded just right.

"One more thing," I said to John. "I want his middle name to be Michael, after St. Michael."

"Michael it is." John knew I wanted the added protection of a guardian angel for our son. This belief that a spiritual being would protect him reassured me. I mentally checked off another box of all the things to do on our road called Perfection Path. I marvelled over sublime thoughts of our future on this path and couldn't wait to see more.

* * *

Countless friends and relatives came to visit after Giaci's birth. They cooed over him.

"He's so precious!"

"Look at that face!"

"No, look at his hands!"

They also overwhelmed us with gifts for baby Giaci. One particular gift stood out. I pulled a child's hockey jersey out of a gift bag, with *Miceli* stamped on the back. The message was clear: Giaci would be an athlete like his father, who played football and basketball. When I looked over at John, I could see that he was already savouring the idea of a life with an athletic son.

John brought up the size of Giaci's hands.

"Look at these," he said, gently grabbing them. "They're big and wide like my dad's! He's gonna dominate in football, you'll see!" he boasted as I nodded in agreement. "Ri, I can't wait to show him how to throw a ball."

Like me, John hungrily anticipated a golden future for his son. We both relished thoughts of him growing, playing sports, and perhaps starring on the varsity team one day—like his father had.

Our happily-ever-after was in the palms of our hands.

As I left the living room to put Giaci to sleep in his bassinet, Lauren was by my side, eager to help. She had already claimed Giaci as her own. Even at her first visit in the hospital, Lauren was protective of her little brother.

When John first brought her to the hospital to see us, they walked into my room hand-in-hand. John, a big man who stood over six feet tall, took sizable strides while Lauren skipped alongside him, trying to keep up in her burgundy turtleneck and black corduroy pants. I could hear part of their conversation as they entered my hospital room.

"—get to see your little brother. Here is Mommy's room."

When they appeared, Lauren practically danced in her slip-on shoes, barely containing herself. Her body jiggled with glee. Her eyes went straight to me in the hospital bed, holding Giaci swaddled in a baby-blue blanket. We both couldn't stop staring at him. With curious eyes, Lauren smiled and asked giddily if she could hold him.

"Mommy, I can do it! I will hold the baby," she affirmed, rubbing her hands together as if to wipe them clean. Lauren was still a baby herself, newly out of diapers, and yet she stood up high on her tippytoes ready to be the baby's second mama.

John swiftly scooped her up and placed her on the bed next to me so she could get a closer look.

We both spotted her as she embraced her little brother for the first time. Lauren moved slowly, wrapping her tiny arms around him like the greatest big sister in the world. She held him gently and safely, making sure her complete, undivided attention was on Giaci.

She looked up at me for a split second, not wanting to spend too much time looking away from the baby. She studied my reaction, expecting me to protest. She was only eighteen months old herself, but it was apparent that Lauren would watch over him and protect him always.

"Okay, *Bella*. Your baby." As soon as I said this, she sighed with relief. She would soon embrace her maternal instincts.

Now at home, as Giaci's little eyes fluttered shut in his bassinet, I could see Lauren peeking in through the door, whispering, "My baby." It warmed and lifted my heart.

When Giaci was asleep, Lauren was like an off-duty mom. The two of us enjoyed our alone time before she went to bed. Looking at both of my sleeping babies, I couldn't believe the great fortune life had offered me. I had two miracles. Two lives prospering.

For months I watched them both hit milestones with ease. Within weeks of coming home from the hospital, Giaci cooed and laughed as he watched his sister dance around him. After only six months he was babbling to Lauren, and she answered him in full sentences. Based on their jovial smiles and energetic movements, it seemed like each one understood what the other was saying. At eight months, Giaci was already walking. It was no surprise to me, as I watched his physical strength and coordination grow almost daily.

Then, suddenly, we noticed a change in Giaci.

SIX

A Fierce Panic

Soon it was Giaci's first birthday. I recalled that, by the time she was one year old, Lauren was already putting up her index finger to indicate her age. She was saying words and interacting with everyone. I realized that Giaci wasn't doing any of this. Why?

I considered this for a few moments, trying to pinpoint anything I may have noticed in his behaviour over the last few days. I felt a familiar worry creep in and decided to hush it rather than give in to it.

He's a boy, I told myself. *Boys are usually later to develop.* That's what my brother David told me when I mentioned the difference between my children. David didn't have any children of his own yet, but he had been around enough children to know there was a difference in how boys and girls developed. I shrugged the whole issue off; I was just too tired.

As the days passed, I tried to maintain a blissful point of view, skipping through life as an overly effervescent woman. But Giaci became increasingly agitated. He cried more and more and was often sluggish. He still wasn't sleeping well, and he often stared into space. He wasn't as happy as he had been as an infant; his cheerful demeanour was dissipating and an inattentive, tired, and downcast child arose. These were definite signs that were cause for concern.

My chest grew tight with worry for my son. It became hard to breathe at times as the nagging, piercing pain in the pit of my stomach persisted. I tried to push it away, thinking that my bubbly, happy baby would return. My anxiety made me queasy.

Whenever Nonna Carolina held him as an infant, she always commented that Giaci was *"bravo e sempre calmo,"* good and always calm. She observed his subdued temperament; he never used to fuss. Was she noticing something? At the time, I thought this was an indication of him being observant and insightful. Now, though, she only commented on how fussy he was.

"What's wrong? Why Giaci cry?"

Looking at the baby in front of me and seeing Giaci squeeze his hands together constantly, my mother's intuition rang out. The alarm in my head screeched. In a haze, I walked to the kitchen, my head rushing through various comparisons between Lauren and Giaci. Of course they would be different, but there seemed to be more to it than the simple differences between individuals. These seemed like clear signs that something was wrong.

I just didn't understand why Giaci wasn't hitting all his developmental milestones like Lauren had. I had raised them the same way.

I turned to the books I'd read about children's growth and development, but they only set off an even fiercer panic. *Childhood Speech, Language, and Listening Problems: What Every Parent Should Know*, by Patricia McAleer Hamaguchi, detailed all the ways in which a toddler should be showing growth in receptive, expressive and social language. I continued reading.

Another book warned that a toddler demonstrating delayed speech or limited use of gestures such as giving, showing, waving, clapping, pointing, or nodding could be cause for concern.

I thought back on all the times we played; Giaci wasn't exhibiting any of these behaviours. He wasn't engaging in play with me. His expression was stoic. He was just there physically, not socially or emotionally.

Yet another book cautioned that if a toddler made odd sounds, had difficulty making or maintaining eye contact, used few gestures or words and showed little or no interest in pretend play, he or she may need to be seen by a professional. This book also mentioned repetitive behaviours and restricted interests, such as lining objects up or repeating words and actions over and over again.

Since turning one, Giaci could spend countless hours rewinding the tapes in the video cassette recorder, watching the same five-minute clip repeatedly, as if he had never seen it before. He would flap his hands and run back and forth all the time, even when I stood in his way to block this never-ending routine.

After all the reading I did, I realized that his behaviour was not the norm. I wondered how I hadn't addressed it sooner. I felt blindsided and knew I had to take matters into my own hands.

I started calling family doctors and pediatricians, making appointment after appointment, hoping to get some answers. After every appointment my mind was spinning, dissatisfied as each doctor tried to put my worries to rest.

"My son didn't talk until he was three, and he's fine now!" one doctor said, patting Giaci on the head.

The next complimented Giaci and dismissed my concerns yet again.

"He's healthy and energetic," he said, barely looking my son. "I don't see any signs for concern. If you're still worried in a year, we can reassess."

Every single doctor made me feel like I was overreacting, and I wanted to believe them. Despite the nagging catastrophic thoughts lingering in the back of my mind and manifesting in the depths of my stomach, I longed for him to be okay. I was torn. My heart didn't want to hear what my head was telling me.

For days, I watched his every move and took notes. Giaci wasn't even making eye contact anymore. I kept begging him to talk to us, but he was more silent than before.

"Giaci, look at me! Look at me, baby boy!"

"Please, Giaci look at me!"

He didn't. He looked everywhere but at me.

My observations just made me tense up more.

When John came home from work one day, I asked him if he'd seen what Giaci had done lately. "He keeps running in circles and will not look at me. He won't engage in play. He just keeps doing things over and over, like obsessing over videos or repetitively jumping on the spot. It doesn't seem right." My voice quavered.

I knew John was overtired from his long hours at work and didn't want to have a conversation about my hypersensitive thoughts, but I was stuck alone with the kids all day. My worries had nowhere else to go. John just looked at me with his soothing eyes and brushed my shoulder gently. "There's nothing to worry about," he said. I couldn't tell if he was just saying this to quiet me or if he genuinely didn't believe anything was wrong with our son. With John, it was sometimes hard to tell the difference.

The days went by, and soon Giaci was eighteen months old. He cried nonstop and I didn't know why. His needs were met. I tried to engage him with kisses, smiles, hugs and playing peek-a-boo. But he still would not reciprocate. He became picky in his eating habits. He limited his food intake to only cereal, milk, and French fries, even though we tried to encourage him with a variety of other foods. He just wouldn't bite.

Despite John's lack of worry, I decided to enrol Giaci in a speech program in the hope that he would acquire more language. I also registered for a parents' program to help teach me how to pull more language out of him; I was willing to do this work alongside him. I would do whatever it took to get him where he needed to be. However, both programs had long waitlists.

"John, I don't want to wait to get some help."

John looked at me, confused because he didn't know what we could do about the waitlists.

"I think we need to enrol him in a daycare so he can be around other children." I waited for John to respond.

"Okay," he said, "if you think this is needed."

This plan of action was new to us, and with anything new came unknowns. Would having Giaci in daycare help ease my fears and concerns? I wasn't sure, but we had to try something.

John and I agreed to enrol him in a specialized daycare centre with a special education resource teacher. The number of children per adult were five to one, which meant he would get more attention. Until now, he had only spent time with his sister, as my mother and John's mother took turns watching the kids while John worked, and I was working half days.

Regardless of whether I could comprehend the realities of our life, we continued daily trying to improve Giaci's communication skills.

"Force the interactions," the special education resource teacher told me. "Do not give him anything unless he verbalizes it."

This was difficult because he didn't verbalize much.

"Put things up high on a shelf so that he points to them."

It all felt repetitive, but I took each bit of advice in hopes of prompting a change. Nothing helped. No matter how high I planted an item, Giaci either ignored or forgot about it. What did he want, and what was he willing to do for it? Why wasn't anything working? Was it me? Was he holding out on me?

As a teacher, when the school year ended, I was excited when the summer arrived. Yet this summer, being at home with the kids all day left me feeling unsettled and alone. Giaci was twenty months old, and he functioned as a six-month-old in socio-emotional development. I was shaken by worrisome thoughts that couldn't go anywhere and were not validated by anyone around me. I was frustrated and, day after day, my uneasiness became worse.

In fact, early morning nausea was becoming a regular thing. I moved slower and tired easily. As I was getting sick in the bathroom one morning, I thought about all the symptoms I was having, and it hit me. I recognized this overwhelming queasiness.

This can't be happening, I thought. *There's no way I could be pregnant.*

SEVEN

"He'll Catch Up, Right?"

No matter how much I tried to will it away, the nausea would not retreat. Finally, after three weeks, I went to the doctor, and she said the words I would have once been thrilled to hear: "You're pregnant! Congratulations."

Fear, worse than what I'd experienced with Lauren, began to creep in. I was scared that this baby would be delayed, like Giaci. I feared not being able to help Giaci and having a new baby to care for. I was scared for her—sweet Lauren, who was already so patient and helpful while we worked through everything with her brother.

Lauren had just turned three and she had taken to the role of the responsible older sister. She never took her eyes off her brother and was always making sure he was safe. She was aware of how fast he could dart off, and so she often held onto him with both hands to keep tabs on him. As little as she was, she was my biggest helper.

Life was flying by without any signs of slowing down, yet paranoid thoughts of an unknown future weighed me down in the never-ending moment. I moved like a robot through daily tasks without much thought or emotion. It was a hazy way to live.

I kept up with my motherly duties, trying to keep a clear head. John would be up early, giving me a peck on the cheek as he ran out the door at six, saying, "Bye, honey!"

Lethargic from pregnancy, I slid out of bed to prepare breakfast for the kids. It was summer break, so I didn't have to go to work until

September. I was falling behind on the household chores and had to entertain two little ones. Not having to go to school made it a bit easier, and as the kids played during the day, I wondered when the speech program waiting list would open up. In the meantime, I tried to implement all the suggestions I gathered.

My strategy was to create learning opportunities to ignite more language use. Since Giaci had a knack for spelling words, I labelled everything in the house. There were words on large cue cards on various items: *clock, fridge, door*, and many more. We had circle time, singing songs to encourage repetition. I set up situations that would force him to interact, like standing in his way and waiting for him to say "Move," or waiting for him to say "Help me" when he needed to put on his shoes. But chasing around an active, rambunctious almost-two-year-old while also trying to engage and pull language out of him was arduous work.

John came home from work each day exhausted, but I was equally exhausted with my stay-at-home job.

Since my attention was squarely on Giaci all day, every day, his delays consumed me. It was all I could think of. John was not obsessed with our son's every move like I was. He didn't see the severity of the situation like I did.

"Rita, don't stress. He'll start talking more soon. Just give it time," he would say each night before bed. His words of advice didn't do me any good, though. They didn't calm me or quiet my racing thoughts. When he turned off the lights, I was still wide awake, trying to think up potential teaching moments for the following day.

I had never imagined that this would be what my life would look like. I had married the love of my life and had two beautiful children, with another on the way, and yet I felt so alone. A numbness wormed its way into my spirit, trying to find a home within me. Sleep didn't come easily for several reasons, and one of them was that Giaci had terrible sleep habits. He was up all night, jumping, making noises, and he did not sleep much. I was up with him a lot. Even when he did doze off, my mind would race for hours with fearful thoughts of an isolated life for my son. If he couldn't interact and communicate with others, how would he make friends? I felt that I was falling short as a mother because I wasn't able to catch him up to his peers.

Giaci was in daycare three days a week when his special education resource teacher suggested taking him to see a psychologist because he wasn't developing like other children. It took months to get an appointment with a private psychologist, and with the wait my anxiety mounted. This particular psychologist had extensive experience assessing and diagnosing patients with learning disabilities, behavioural problems, and adaptation problems, but could she help Giaci? Would she know what was wrong with him?

John held an almost-two-year-old Giaci as we walked into her office. Half-moon-shaped shadows hung beneath my eyes. I was teaching full-time that school year and was exhausted by the thought of this entire process. Her office was pristine and orderly, with books shelved by size and colour and papers arranged in piles. I could feel my anxiety shifting into irritation as I studied her gold-rimmed glasses that sat on her aquiline nose. I was irritated by the fact of having to be there, by having to go through this process. *Why is this happening to us? It shouldn't be.*

Giaci squirmed his hand out of John's grip, trying to run away, so John put Giaci on his lap. John's expression was calm and at ease. He still didn't acknowledge the possibility that his son needed more support than many other children typically did. I held the arm rest of my chair tightly as I braced myself for what was about to be said.

Dr. Helen began to ask question after question. "Does he point? Does he make eye contact? Does he engage in play? Does he like to be touched?" These were questions that I had already answered many times before with other professionals. It was like being hit repeatedly on an open wound.

I answered her questions, one after another, while John held Giaci firmly as he persistently tried to squirm out of John's arms. "No, he doesn't. No, he doesn't do that either. No, he can't do that. No, he doesn't." It was a gruelling interrogation, and my fingernails were cutting the palms of my hand as I gripped the arm rest tighter.

This went on for about an hour. "I'd like to observe your son in the play area in the next room," the psychologist said. So we brought Giaci over and she observed from behind a two-way mirror, taking notes on her clipboard with her sharp pencil.

After about twenty minutes, she came into the room where we were with Giaci. "This concludes our appointment today," she said.

She didn't apologize for the waitlist, nor did she seem concerned about my obvious anxiety. I imagined she was looking at my almost-five-months-along pregnant belly and wondering how a mother like me could possibly handle another one. I brushed the thought away and continued listening.

"Once I've completed the summary of his assessment, I'll look over the results, and then we can meet to discuss everything." She seemed almost cheery with her nonchalant approach. For her, my family's phone number was just another data point on a long list. It was as if we'd taken a number at the deli, and she was eager to give us our order and get us out the door before her next customer.

Almost a month passed before she called us back to her office to deliver her diagnosis. The calm look on her face didn't match the news she gave us. "Giaci has PDD—pervasive developmental disorder." She gave it to us straight. I had never heard of this. My face and John's must have looked stunned because she waited a beat before continuing. "In short, he's developmentally delayed."

"A delay means he'll catch up, right?" I blurted out. A delay didn't seem so bad. Trains were delayed all the time, but they still got to their destinations.

"Yes, that is the hope. But he will need interventions to catch up. I would start by getting a speech pathologist working with him," she answered.

Her report didn't contain any additional diagnoses, so when she reached the end of her sheet, I settled back in my chair, relieved. John looked over at me as if to say *I told you so*. We both felt like we'd dodged a bullet. It could have been worse; a delay we could deal with.

When we got home that evening, I made a new game plan to get Giaci up to speed. I would contact a speech pathologist first so they could get started right away. John put the kids to bed while I planned. To ease my racing mind and calm the churning in my growing belly, I took to the internet to search for strategies and ideas on how to pull more language out of my son.

I came across the fourth edition of the *Diagnostic and Statistical Manual of Mental Disorders*, or DSM-IV, which was the standard manual used by mental health professionals to classify mental disorders.

In Part A of one set of diagnostic criteria, the DSM-IV indicated that if a child had "a total of six (or more) items from (1), (2) and (3), with at least two from (1) and one each from (2) and (3)," then the child had Autistic Disorder:

(1) Qualitative impairments in social interaction, as manifested by at least two of the following:

(a) marked impairments in the use of multiple nonverbal behaviors such as eye-to-eye gaze, facial expression, body posture, and gestures to regulate social interaction

(b) failure to develop peer relationships appropriate to developmental level

(c) a lack of spontaneous seeking to share enjoyment, interests, or achievements with other people (e.g., by a lack of showing, bringing, or pointing out objects of interest to other people)

(2) Qualitative impairments in communication as manifested by at

least one of the following:

(a) delay in, or total lack of, the development of spoken language (not accompanied by an attempt to compensate through alternative modes of communication such as gesture or mime)

(b) in individuals with adequate speech, marked impairment in the ability to initiate or sustain a conversation with others

(c) stereotyped and repetitive use of language or idiosyncratic language

(d) lack of varied, spontaneous make-believe play or social imitative play appropriate to developmental level

(3) Restricted repetitive and stereotyped patterns of behavior, interests, and activities, as manifested by at least two of the following:

(a) encompassing preoccupation with one or more stereotyped and restricted patterns of interest that is abnormal either in intensity or focus

(b) apparently inflexible adherence to specific, non-functional routines or rituals

(c) stereotyped and repetitive motor mannerisms (e.g., hand or finger flapping or twisting, or complex whole-body movements)

(d) persistent preoccupation with parts of objects

As if that wasn't enough, there was a part B:

B. Delays or abnormal functioning in at least one of the following areas, with onset prior to age 3 years:

(1) social interaction;

(2) language as used in social communication;

(3) symbolic or imaginative play

There was also something called Asperger's Disorder, and the non-specific Pervasive Developmental Disorder Not Otherwise Specified.

As I read through the DSM-IV, I mentally checked off all the items of these lists that applied to my son. I tallied up my mental checkmarks: Giaci had almost everything on it.

My heart seized up.

The tears gushed as if a storm cloud had burst. I gripped the edge of my chair, feeling lightheaded. All the moisture in my mouth vanished. This new possibility rendered me motionless. I didn't know anyone who had an autistic child, nor did I know anything about autism.

Despite the professionals we were dealing with—the family doctors, the pediatricians, the resource teacher, and now the psychologist—no one had ever mentioned the word *autism*. It hadn't even been on my radar, and now my brain was trying to catch up. I felt like I was struggling through the last few minutes of a test that I was sure to fail.

What did *autism* even mean? I'd seen the movie *Rain Man*; would my son be like Dustin Hoffman's character, Raymond Babbitt? The thought sent me into a scrolling frenzy, searching for other answers, searching for a mislabelling or a Wikipedia sense of falsehood. While my eyes scanned the screen, my brain reviewed various conversations with the different family doctors and pediatricians. Did even one of them mention autism? Did I just block them out? My brain kept asking questions that I didn't have the answers to.

I stumbled up the stairs to tell John. I couldn't sit on this alone. But when I got to the top of the stairs, I broke down right at the edge. I struggled to find the air to breathe; I had to get to John. I hurried to our bedroom to find that he was already in bed. His eyes were closed but he wasn't in a deep sleep. I nudged him. This couldn't wait.

When he opened his eyes, he noticed my crumbling state. He sat up, asking, "What's wrong?"

I couldn't say the word anywhere except in my head, and even that was a stretch. I couldn't speak. I just led him back downstairs and pointed to the computer screen. When I saw his face, I knew that he had registered what I had. The pain consumed us both inside a bubble.

At least John was inside the bubble with me now.

EIGHT

Why My Son?

Giaci was falling further and further behind, and he was increasingly living in his own world. He watched clips of animated videos repeatedly, rewinding them, and then watching them yet again. He flapped his hands vigorously while jumping in place in front of the television. I'd sit on the sofa behind him, watching and wondering where his mind and thoughts had disappeared to. Lauren played in the room behind me with her stuffed toys, pretending they were her girlfriends. She was almost three and a half now, and held elaborate conversations with her imaginary friends, discussing her favourite ice cream and her pretty outfit.

Why? Why? Why MY son? The words beat to the rhythm of every mundane activity around the house. Feeding, dressing, and teaching were still on the agenda, and I couldn't let my children down more than I already had. Everything I did always felt like it was never enough because Giaci was not improving. Every time I buried myself in darkness, I had to pull myself out of it for Lauren, Giaci, and the new arrival.

We were now four months away from welcoming a new Miceli, and my anticipation wasn't like the nervousness I'd felt with Lauren or the excitement with Giaci; it was pure numbness, clean and detached. What had happened to my happily ever after? I'd always envisioned that John and I would have a big family, and now we were getting exactly what we'd hoped for. I beat myself up for not being more excited. *This is what you wanted, Rita. Isn't it?*

But the vision I'd once held now felt hazy and tainted. It wasn't what I had expected from my perfect life: John was always working, Giaci was in his own world, and Lauren was stuck with a shell of a mother who slipped away to cope when her daughter needed her most.

My eyes were half open, and I was unable to see clearly. My energy was depleted by lack of sleep, and I was emotionally depleted from all the worry and anxiety that consumed me. I was a mere shadow of myself.

John handled stress differently than I did; it was the result of my emotional brain versus his logical brain. Italian men were taught to be strong, not weak. When faced with a crisis, he suppressed his emotions and dove into work, whereas I was driven by emotions, which often thrust me into fight-or-flight mode. I expressed the fight with anger, and the flight was my depressive state, when I was in darkness.

My belly was growing exponentially by the second. I remember commenting to John, "I feel much bigger this time."

I thought that maybe going in for my ultrasound would bring joy back into my life and make me feel like it was worth living again. I had asked to hold off on the ultrasound until it would show the baby's sex, hoping this would calm my nerves a bit; at that time, four out of five children diagnosed with autism were boys.

John took the day off work to come with me, but we didn't dare talk about Giaci or the concern we shared. Our newfound realization was still fermenting, and we functioned like automatons.

At the medical building, John stayed in the waiting room with Giaci and Lauren. As soon as I lay on the bed, the technician began recording images. She was young and didn't say much; I could only assume it was because she was focused on what she was doing. My thoughts raced. *Will this child be a girl like Lauren, or a boy like Giaci? Girl or boy?* After several minutes of silence, the technician paused and said, "Turn more to your right, please. I've finished one baby."

I started to turn, then froze and stared at her, confused by her comment.

"What do you mean, 'one baby'? Do you want me to get the next mom in line?" I asked.

"No," she said. "I meant that I've finished taking images of one of your babies—this one is a girl—and now I'm going to do your second baby."

My mouth dropped open. "You might want to call your supervisor. I think there must be some mistake," I said, feeling a tsunami of tears arriving.

The technician asked, "Would you like me to call your husband in?"

I nodded, sobbing. It felt like I was drowning without a flotation device in sight.

John entered the room holding Giaci in his arms. Lauren walked closely beside him. He saw me crying and asked, "What's wrong, Rita? You okay?"

After a pause, not knowing how to answer, I simply said, "No."

"Why? What's going on?" John asked, confused by my agitated state.

"We are having *twins!*" I wailed.

His reaction was not what I was expecting. He gazed at me with a smile. But it was a cautious smile.

John was excited by the news. He wanted many children and was confident we would be okay because of the love we had for one another. I was terrified at the prospect of having four young children at home. And part of me still had hope in God's plan for us; maybe God knew we needed these extra teammates to help with Giaci's care. I mirrored John's cautious smile. It was the first time I had felt something other than sorrow in months.

Before going home, we headed to John's parents' house. They wanted to hear if we were having a boy or a girl. As we drove, I realized that we hadn't even asked about the second baby's sex. I was still in a state of shock. So many thoughts were racing through my mind. *How will I be able to continue working? How will I care for two more babies and help Giaci?* My head was spinning, and I was trapped in a whirlwind of emotions.

When we arrived, John's family was sitting at the kitchen table waiting to hear our news. My eyes were glossy, and my mother-in-law noticed the visible signs that I had been crying.

"What's wrong?" she asked.

I couldn't get the words out, so John jumped in and said, "It's great news, Mom. We're having twins!"

After a brief pause in which everyone processed the news, there was an eruption of excitement. Well wishes of "Congratulations!" and "That's awesome!" echoed around us. John's siblings and parents buzzed around us excitedly, talking about how amazing it was that *two* more Micelis were coming into this world. I watched all their delighted faces and saw how John was beginning to echo their excitement, but I still couldn't muster up a confident smile. I stood frozen with fear, trying my best to hide it from everyone else. I didn't dare tell them why I was upset or that all I could think about was the possibility of the twins being like Giaci.

How was I supposed to break the news about Giaci to all these thrilled faces? I kept trying to swallow my worry, but it just wouldn't go down. I hoped that no one would notice and that the worry would eventually disappear.

It did not.

NINE

A Race Against Time

The solitude crept in. Those first wintry days, I felt buoyed by my grade 6 students, who displayed an eager holiday spirit. At school my students were enthusiastic, keen to learn and to interact with me and with one other. My colleagues and I worked as a team; there was a unified approach to attain the curriculum expectations. Meanwhile, at home I was alone, teaching through a thick maritime fog. There was no view of colourful seaside houses, no directions to help me sail home; it was just me paddling in circles, trying to find my way to shore.

When I got home after a long day of teaching, my compass led me straight to the computer to search for more answers for what was happening for Giaci. Part of me knew that I had the answer, but a large part of me wasn't ready to fully acknowledge the diagnosis. If I acknowledged it, I was admitting weakness and powerlessness in the face of this disability that was draining the life from me.

I couldn't yet wave the flag of failure or admit the loss of my perfect world. If I could find a solution—a *cure*—maybe I would never have to tell anyone about Giaci because he'd be better. As far as I was concerned, it was my job to make him better, to cure him.

On one website I read that by the time a child is two years old, a diagnosis by an experienced professional is considered reliable. However, many children do not receive a final diagnosis until they are older. It was clear from everything I read that the earlier the diagnosis, the sooner treatment could begin. And the sooner treatment could begin, the better the child's life outcomes would be. *The better our lives and Giaci's will be*, I thought.

As soon as I read this, the button on my internal stopwatch was pressed, and the intense ticking of the timer vibrated emphatically in my ears. Every minute was valuable treatment time that we could not afford to lose.

We were now in a race against time, and this race would determine how Giaci's life would unfold.

Giaci was only two, but the guilt of not having stepped in sooner consumed me. Even though I still couldn't say the word *autism*, I needed to forge ahead with a plan.

If I acted now, everything might be normal by the time the twins arrived. We'd be prepared, and we could get our lives back on track.

TEN

The Wrestling Game

Soon, I realized that getting back on track might not be easy or smooth.

"*That's* why he isn't interacting with us—he is in pain," I said when John and I finally learned about Giaci's baby-bottle-induced tooth decay. The pediatric dentist informed us that Giaci would need surgery for the cavities he had in his front teeth.

At the hospital, Giaci was sedated. The pediatric dentist dulled a nerve connected to his front teeth, treated the tooth decay, and then placed crowns over the affected teeth, which blended in perfectly with his other teeth. Giaci appeared even more adorable with his full shiny set of pearly whites.

After the dental surgery, he started eating more. He still stuck to a limited selection of foods, but he did not cry as much. Although he never slept through the night, Giaci did seem happier. This was the bright light I needed; maybe this had been the real reason for his delayed speech, and now everything would move forward as usual.

Still, John and I continued to not bring up his diagnosis. We didn't dare acknowledge our son's delays, although they glared at us daily. Instead, I clung to the hope that it was all a terrible mistake. I knew this was a hope flickering in John's eyes too.

We both longed to hear Giaci speak. We would sit with him and Lauren each evening, hoping that if he didn't communicate with *us*, maybe Lauren could pull words out of him.

At bedtime, with Lauren and Giaci tucked into the sheets, I would grab a Dr. Seuss book and read it to them. Lauren always paid attention and asked questions, but Giaci preferred to study his fingers as he wiggled them oddly close to his eyes. Lauren didn't question her brother's limitations or odd behaviour because that was all she knew; it was normal to her. Instead, she would physically push his hands down and manoeuvre his face, forcing him to look at the book. Her understanding of her brother's abilities and the patience with which she conducted herself were greater than what most adults possessed.

One evening, I struggled to produce a smile as I watched Lauren engage with her brother in any way she could. She was wise and could identify my seesaw of emotions beneath my surface-level grin.

"Mommy, Giaci will learn to read to me one day. I know it!" she said with such purity in her voice. "We'll teach him how, right?"

I nodded in agreement and kissed them both on the forehead, saying, "Good night. Love you."

Lauren answered, "Good night. Love you, Mommy. Love you, Giaci." With that, she rolled over to face her brother in the queen-sized bed they shared, wrapping her arm around him as he lay silently beside her.

So often, I could see progress in Giaci, like the time he ran up to me and pointed to the cereal box he wanted. But then, the next minute, that progress ground to a halt and I couldn't figure out what he wanted. It was like he didn't have enough words to express himself. He was now verbalizing a few words, like *Daddy* and *Mommy*, but I had an insatiable thirst for more. I desperately wanted to hear him say, "I love you, Mommy."

Repeating the words *Mommy* and *Daddy*, paired with pointing at me and John, was what I did constantly. It was like a recording on repeat. Over and over I said it, whenever I had his attention. And then one day, at the dinner table, Giaci heard Lauren say, "Mommy, a cup please," and for the first time, Giaci said, "Mommy." I froze with a smile, then burst into cheers. He smiled back at me. Before long, it was an ongoing regular occurrence. He said, "Mommy," and I would light up. He would enjoy the back and forth. I approached it the same way with "Daddy," and got John involved in the process.

My adrenaline pumped fiercely as Giaci's words came in slowly. I needed help to get more language out of him. John and I were desperate for professional help. Then, when we finally got the call from the speech program, we rejoiced.

A woman called to book our first meeting at the Regional Hospital, not too far from our home in Windsor. "We would like you to come this Monday for an initial meeting at nine o'clock in the morning. Please bring your son's favourite snacks and comfortable clothes, as we may be doing some floor activities." She spoke slowly and enunciated every word. I wrote all the information down, not wanting to miss a thing. "Of course," I replied. "And thank you, thank you so much. We will be there."

After months on the waitlist for the hospital's Early Language Intervention program, we were finally in. In this program, Giaci would receive half-hour, one-to-one sessions once a week for six weeks to train us to help him gain more language. There were also two sessions—one in the middle of the program and one at the end—in which the parents and children did specific activities and interacted together.

John and I were pumped and ready to launch these new strategies into play in hopes of hearing more language from our son.

Elaine was the speech pathologist in charge, and she told us to begin by making Giaci aware of imitation. I had to imitate everything he did. If he ran back and forth, I ran back and forth. If he jumped up and down flapping his hands, I gently hopped up and down flapping my hands.

While I was off work now, per my doctor's advice, I spent my time wisely and devoted my days to imitating a toddler. This feeling of being constantly "on" was exhausting enough in itself; being pregnant with twins while doing so was even harder. I wasn't about to take my eyes off first base, though; first would lead to second, and eventually we would be barreling toward home. I was geared up and ready to do whatever we had to.

Because I was focusing all my time on my son, there wasn't much time for anything else. John worked a lot, and I was always "on" with the kids. Our families noticed changes in our behaviour, as we were harder to reach and constantly seemed distracted. We would be invited to visit with my parents or John's, but we would often decline, saying that I was too tired due to the pregnancy, or that John was too busy with work. Our excuses were valid, so no one questioned us. The truth was that we had little energy to focus on anything else.

Since Giaci's PDD diagnosis, we hadn't told anyone the full story. The word *autism* wasn't clearly laid out in the documents, even though we now knew that they were one and the same. We were too worried that family and friends wouldn't understand the extent of Giaci's problems or how difficult it was for John and me, especially since Giaci was not progressing as rapidly as we hoped. This fear muted us, making the reality difficult to talk about.

When we did attend family gatherings, we both found them exhausting. Explaining Giaci's condition to a half-listening audience over a plate of meatballs and broccoli dip was simply too draining. But somehow, the act of pretending everything was fine was worse.

When Giaci flapped his hands, I would stop him by holding his hands and redirect him elsewhere, away from anyone. When Giaci mumbled inaudible sounds, I would pretend like he really said something, "Oh, okay Giaci, we can go to the bathroom." Meanwhile, it was all just creative nonfiction, and I was just ad-libbing.

It was nearly impossible to break free of the helplessness I felt in dealing with Giaci's struggles. I was living a life that was half in my head and half outside it, constantly pretending that everything was okay. Drained and frustrated that no one could hear the screaming in my head, I occasionally wondered if this was what Giaci was experiencing. We both wanted to be understood, to communicate fully with the world, but were unable to do so.

Every time I opened my mouth to share the diagnosis with family members, I automatically diverted the conversation to the twins' upcoming birth. I felt the need to keep the positivity going and to not let anyone in on the cloud of uncertainty surrounding us. We were going through the fatigue-induced motions, unsure of what our next move was. The twins seemed like a safe place to land, a beacon of hope.

But these pent-up emotions needed to come out, and the safest place for that to happen was in the shower. I didn't want anyone to hear me. I didn't dare show my family that I was falling apart. What would others think? What kind of mother would that make me? The sound of the water masked my uncontrollable sobbing. As the tears trickled down my face, they lingered on my wet lips and tasted salty, like the sea.

One day, my crying transformed into anger. I was helpless, and it felt insurmountable. I realized that something had to give. I had to abandon my career ambitions. My life wasn't my own anymore.

I allowed myself to grieve in the shower, knowing the moment I stepped out, I had to own my decision. After the twins arrived, I wouldn't go back to full-time work. My children's well-being was more important, and I had to step into the role of full-time mother.

When I got out of the shower, I shared my decision with John.

"John," I called out, wrapping myself in a towel. He was settling into bed with the television on, just seconds away from changing the channel and tuning out the world altogether. I waited until he looked over at me before telling him about my decision to only work part-time after the six-month maternity leave I had after the twins were born.

His reaction was exactly what I expected. "Rita, I understand, and if that's what you want to do, that's fine. I think that's what's best for our family right now, but that doesn't mean it always has to be this way. Things may change." John considered the facts and processed them like an equation. Just like with Giaci's symptoms, he calculated the $a + b = c$ of what it meant for me to be home more. It would mean he would need to take on additional work to be able to financially provide for the support that Giaci needed.

* * *

As John worked longer and longer hours—often until well into the evening—the brunt of the child-rearing work fell increasingly to me. Still, every day before changing into his construction gear to go to his other job, he always made time to play with Giaci.

During this playtime, Giaci just seemed like every other little boy in the world. John would hoist him in the air over his head and onto his shoulders. He then tickled him and wrestled him onto the couch cushions.

As John lifted Giaci, their pearly white smiles brightened their faces, and they radiated excitement and rambunctious camaraderie. When John released Giaci, Giaci's hair flew back and the skin on his face smoothed out from the pressure of the air before he crashed into the leather cushions. As he landed, Giaci loosed a high-pitched squeak. Father and son roared with laughter, like a lion with his cub, and they wore the biggest smiles as they re-enacted an episode of the World Wrestling Championships.

Seeing them both enjoy these special moments felt like a warm blanket settling over my shoulders. I envied the horseplay. I carried all the weight of dealing with Giaci's condition, but none of the glory. I tried to settle for the role of entertained observer, but I was jealous of John's connection with our son. I hadn't found a similar connector yet. My role of being his mother meant I was his teacher, his guide, and the person who would always push him to work harder. John enjoyed his time with our son, and I had the all-work-and-no-play state of mind.

My connection with Lauren came through conversation, and I desperately longed to bond the same way with Giaci. I wished I could know what he was thinking and have a conversation about his likes and dislikes.

Then, as I watched them wrestle one day, it clicked. I could become involved in their game by inserting teaching moments in the play wrestling. Like a coach on the sidelines, I told John to wait on the release of his body slam until Giaci said "Go!"

The first time, John and I modelled it. Then, Giaci started to repeat the word to get the desired response: being spiritedly slammed down onto the cushions. Soon, they were both following this format without any reminders from me. Whenever Giaci wanted a body slam, he would go up to John and say "Go!" or "Go, Daddy!" Soon enough, it had stretched to "I want wrestle, Daddy!" My cheers roared from the sidelines, as this game seemed to be the greatest motivation for his words. I was hungry for more from Giaci, and now I knew how to draw language from him.

They continued to play this game almost every day, even allowing Lauren to jump in. As I watched, I saw how Lauren served as a role model for her brother. She would add more words, like "Do it again, Daddy!" and Giaci would try to imitate her, even though his words weren't as clear as Lauren's.

He beamed with each throwdown and expressed himself by squeezing his palms together and stiffening his legs before he released his words. He seemed to enjoy the pressure on his little body as he flew through the air. It motivated him to communicate, and I encouraged these moments because I wanted to hear him say "I love you."

Whenever John held Lauren in the air above his head, I would clearly say, "I love you, Lauren," to which she would respond, "I love you, Mommy! Go, Daddy!" Only after that would she be catapulted into the air and then engulfed by the sofa.

Giaci watched, laughing hysterically, and then we would do the same action with him. Then, finally, one day we heard the words I longed to hear.

Giaci said, "Wuv you, Mommy." My heart soared. I could have listened to him say those words all day. To most mothers, this was a natural expression that might be taken for granted. For me, this was everything.

John stared at me, seeing my delight. The wrestling with verbal cues continued.

Now Giaci knew that he had to use his words to play this game; otherwise, the wrestling moves would stop. Once the words were said, an explosion of sensory experiences ensued. It was sensory food that Giaci hungered for, and his actions produced a reaction that was teaching him all about interaction. We could see the power in what motivated Giaci.

Now, multiple times a day, the words *I love you* were said among the four of us.

I love you, Giaci.

I love you, Lauren.

I love you, Daddy.

I love you, Mommy.

"I love you more," I'd always respond.

ELEVEN

A True Puzzle

One day in mid-January, I watched Giaci line up the magnetic letters on the fridge. His little fingers grasped one letter at a time, and he then placed them on the fridge door in rigid lines. I could see that he was putting them together to spell words.

"Good boy, buddy!" I said with pride, as if he had accomplished brain surgery.

I watched him form words and phrases such as *authorized* and *feature presentation* with ease. These were oversized and complex words for a two-year-old. How was this possible? He could spell big words that were beyond the understanding of other children his age, let alone the ability to pronounce them. Yet he couldn't even answer simple questions like "How old are you?" and "What's your name?" He must have seen those more complex words—but where? In a parking lot (*authorized parking*) or in a video (*feature presentation*)? I realized he was remembering the words to spell them.

It was clear that my son's learning was sporadic and didn't follow any sort of building-block sequence. He had pockets of deficits. His cognitive, expressive, receptive and verbal skills may have been delayed, but his visual ability was heightened.

The brain is a complex organ, a true puzzle. I often found myself wondering, *How does his brain work?* If there was a disconnect between different areas of his brain, was there a way to connect the wires to make it all work like it was supposed to? This gave me hope, and I knew that deep down the true Giaci was waiting to be released.

I continued to watch him line up the magnets. What else could he show off?

Most of Giaci's days were spent running back and forth, like the Road Runner from the *Looney Tunes* cartoons. He could do this aimlessly, happily, and repeatedly for hours. Now, after several minutes of spelling out large, complex words, he returned to this activity. It was like lights that flickered on and off, observable from an outside window.

His repetitive behaviours overwhelmed me, and my inability to stop them made me grit my teeth. I could never hold my helplessness in. "Stop running!" I yelled, knowing that it wouldn't do much good. Giaci would stop for a beat, then continue on as he had been.

He lived in his own solitary world and was happy to stay there. Most days, it felt like he didn't even need me. Every time I tried to enter that world with him, fear stopped me at the doors. Since he was happy there, would my interference cause him unhappiness? A solitary life seemed sad, and I longed for him to live in *this* world, with me. I wanted to pull him to the surface. I needed a new tactic. Since yelling didn't work, I needed to redirect my attention to something more productive.

While Giaci continued to run around the living room and kitchen, I opened a drawer and pulled out my teaching cue cards. I began scribbling the word for everything that Giaci came into contact with: *clock, door, bathroom, window, fridge, stove*...the list went on and on. I was in super-teacher mode, hoping for enlightenment but also for a distraction from his repetitive actions.

I couldn't afford to lose even one minute of valuable teaching time because every moment counted. I wanted to see Giaci learning at warp speed because once the twins were born, life would become even more hectic. So, I needed to make the most of this time with my son now, which meant I wasn't as focused on getting the nursery ready or anything else for the twins' arrival as I was during my first two pregnancies.

As soon as the cards were finished and taped up, I walked Giaci and Lauren around the house, hand in little hand, pointing out all the labelled cue cards. Given Giaci's ability to spell, I hoped that seeing these words written out would help him retain more language. Even though these efforts made sense to me, I didn't see any real progress.

There was another area I needed to focus on with Giaci: toilet training. He was still in diapers, and the prospect of having three children in diapers at the same time exhausted me. There was no way of knowing how long it would take to teach this skill, so we had to start right away.

Giaci's ability to respond to "I love you" with an "I love you" of his own remained current. In fact, he was now able to say, "Love you, Mommy." Progress like this energized me, but it also left me pining for more.

Just as quickly as my energy came, though, my sleep deprivation drove it away, making it hard to function. I couldn't shake the belief that I was failing my son by not successfully helping him catch up to his peers, and this kept me awake at night. In addition, Giaci was always up at night running around all over the house, and I was uncomfortable from the twins' rapid growth inside me. We tried a baby gate to keep him in his room, but he would just jump over it. The only solution was for me or John to physically get up and repeatedly bring him back to his bed. This became my new normal and I didn't dare ask anyone for help. How could I? I didn't want anyone to see how Giaci was presenting himself or how I couldn't handle or fulfill my motherly role. Living in denial was easier, and I held on to the hope that his diagnosis would somehow magically disappear.

Despite the lack of sleep we both endured, John still trudged to work each morning. He was conditioned to do so. It's what his father and mine would have done. We'd grown up watching them do whatever it took to put food on our dinner tables and to create opportunity in our lives.

My dad worked hard cutting hair every day, without ever taking a sick day, and then on Sundays he always tended to necessary repairs at the rental properties he owned. John's dad worked the night shifts at an automotive plant and took every bit of overtime that was offered. We didn't see our dads much growing up because they worked all the time.

Like our parents before us, we worked to provide freedom and opportunity for our children. Our version of freedom just looked a little different. Our parents wanted to give us freedom from physical toil; we wanted to give our children mental freedom.

And so, every morning, John looked more and more like his father as he got ready for his day. Exhaustion circled his eyes, and for the first time I noticed our youth escaping us. It was drained by our lifestyle, but it had to be. Without fail, John would try to wash the sleepiness from his eyes before he came back to kiss me goodbye. He always tried to appear stronger, unfazed by our endless go-go-go lifestyle, but after being with him for twelve years, I had learned to reach into those deep pockets where he stashed secrets.

"Have a good day, John," I said one morning as I rolled over. I'd been pretending that I was still asleep until that moment; I couldn't sleep and I didn't want to wake him. As I tried to sit up to take another look at him before he left, he settled back onto the edge of the bed.

"Don't move," he said. "You know what the doctor said." As I rested my hands on my belly, he kissed each hand tenderly, as if kissing both our babies through them.

I heard the doctor's voice echo again in my head: *You're a high-risk pregnancy.* I was already in my fifth month when we found out that we were having twins, and if I hadn't already been nervous about this pregnancy, the doctor's warning would have made me. Due to my "high-risk" status, I was off work and basically homebound.

"Just try not to stress," he added, bringing me back to our moment on the bed. "Rest, relax, and ask your mom or mine for help with the kids today." I nodded, but he wasn't convinced of my compliance. "Promise me? You don't have to do this alone." He kissed me once more before checking the time and dashing out for his full day.

I just couldn't ask for help.

On days like these, I wished we could lie in bed all day without a worry in the world. It was hard to imagine that ever being possible again.

Once upon a time, we were carefree and in love, growing closer and closer and dreaming of our perfect life. Now that was a distant memory; John was barely home, and I was always stressed and exhausted. We hardly communicated with each other. As much as we still had moments of love and devotion, we were like two separate cars on a train—one in front, one in back. We were moving in the same direction, but we were disconnected from each other, with other cars linked between us.

Before rolling out of bed each day, I would stare at the ceiling, hoping that my message to heaven would reach its destination. "Lord," I'd pray, "it's a new day. Please give me the patience I need and grant me the strength to manage." I'd plead with my hands clasped together. Talking to God, the feelings of loneliness and abandonment disappeared for a moment, but as soon as God and I were alone in conversation, I felt the emotional floodgates open. *Why is my son unable to communicate his needs? Why am I struggling to help him understand things? Am I being tested?* My jaw clenched even as my thoughts and feelings released. I couldn't help but interrogate God. I was angry at how difficult life had become.

I was locked in an eternal battle between positive and negative thoughts about my faith. There were moments when I thanked God for helping me through this, but just as quickly, the switch would flip, and I would wonder why God had abandoned me. My anger at this inconsistent God was a constant through my days. It was my new form of prayer—the prayer of a lost and desperate soul. I hated God for making me question Him.

Still, I prayed for answers, for more of a connection with my husband, for more help. I prayed just to be able to get out of bed.

The only driving force in my life was my children. Even though I could barely keep my eyes open due to the struggles of motherhood, my role was also the only motivator getting me through the day. While John was out focusing on the finances, I focused on the kids' survival, and mine. When their wiggling bodies got out of bed, that was my cue.

"Mommy, can we play?" Lauren said as soon as I entered their bedroom, her hair still a tangled curly mess.

"Yes, honey. What do you want to play?" I asked, waddling over to help her out of bed.

"I want to play pretend!" Even this early in the day, she was all smiles.

Soon I was dragging my pregnant body around the house and gathering up all the costumes, hats, and whatever toys Lauren needed to fulfill her very precise early morning tea-party scene. I pulled out the children's table and chairs and laid out a flowy, floral blue, yellow and white oversized dress for Lauren, who would complete the look with my floppy straw hat. For Giaci, I pulled out his white button-down dress shirt and blue dress pants and grabbed an old tie that John never wore. I also had an old-fashioned men's brown fedora that had belonged to my father. With their attire ready, I turned back to Lauren.

"Okay, honey," I said, "I need you to find all your stuffed animals so they can come to your tea party with Giaci! Can you get them out of your playhouse and put them where you want so you can serve them tea too?" Playtime had begun, and my tone had to come along for the ride, a skill I had cultivated in my work as a teacher. Lauren couldn't tell if I was pretending to be okay or if I actually was. What mattered most was that we were playing together.

Lauren calculated who she should invite to her party. Her nose had scrunched up when I suggested some of her stuffy friends. She shook her head, giggling. Still maintaining eye contact, she announced, "It will be me, Giaci, Pink Elephant, and Teddy! We're going to have fun!" She squeaked as she ran to assemble her invited guests, leaving a seat for herself and her brother.

I took out Lauren's toy tea set and then fetched a glass of water to fill their cups. I came back to find Lauren dressed and ready to go. She had also started dressing her brother in his outfit. Giaci was compliant with his bossy big sister. As Lauren took off his T-shirt, she explained to him what was happening.

"Now listen to me. We are going to play teatime, so you have to wear this nice shirt." She dragged her words out to make them clear, in case he missed anything, as she continued to dress him in his "old man" clothing, directing the entire scene.

"And then you're gonna wear Daddy's tie and Nonno's hat. Okay? Giaci, listen to me!" She manoeuvred his arms while pulling his shirt on and then placed the tie over his head and loosely around his neck.

"Giaci, look at me, I'm talking to you."

Giaci didn't seem to listen, but he complied. She didn't give him much of a choice. I smiled while watching the purity of their sibling interaction and placed the water and a few cookies on the table without getting in Lauren's way. Once she had put the fedora on Giaci's head, he was ready for the tea party.

Lauren dragged her submissive guest to the chair, sat him down, and adjusted him so that his legs were under the table. I waddled upstairs to grab my camera, not wanting to miss a bit of this memory. Lauren didn't notice me taking pictures because she was too busy being an incredible host to her little brother and her stuffed toy friends. As she poured the water into the teacups, she jumped into character.

"Now, be careful, Mr. Giaci—this tea is very hot! Ouch! See? Be careful, I said."

His wordless responses seemed to direct their conversation. He participated with a perplexed expression, unable to verbalize what he was thinking, which was fine with Lauren, since she liked to do all the talking anyway. After sitting down in her own little chair, she encouraged him to drink from his teacup.

"Drink it, Giaci! It's deeelishious. You will like it." She placed her petite hands over her brother's equally small hands, manipulating him like he was one of her dolls or stuffed guests. I just stood off to the side, smiling and trying to soak in each minute.

"Okay, friends, it's time for a treat! I have...cookies! Look, Giaci, I have a cookie for you. Here you go!" She tenderly held the plate out to show Giaci the cookies. His eyes opened wide as if he were ready to devour the entire plate. This made the entire dressing up and sitting down process much more bearable for him.

"Now, only take one. Only one," Lauren emphasized, putting her index finger up to make sure he only took one, an instruction he followed.

This beautiful interaction lasted until Giaci finished the cookie—getting what he had wanted from the start—and darted away into the other room to play by himself with his toys. Lauren watched him run but didn't break character. The tea party scene between Lauren and her stuffed toy friends went on for hours.

I couldn't believe Giaci had lasted as long as he did.

Since he was a runner, I could never take my eyes off him, and I followed him into the next room. He moved nonstop, climbing like Spider-Man, bouncing around like a ping-pong ball. Thankfully, when John built the current house, he made sure to install an alarm system. If the door to the outside were opened, I would hear a beep. This meant Giaci couldn't run out of the house without us knowing.

Still, my heart palpitated at the mere thought of losing sight of him. I often struggled to calm myself and wondered how the constant up and down of my heartbeat was affecting the twins.

I took three deep breaths while Giaci entertained himself.

Why hadn't anyone warned me that this was what my motherhood would look like? In these moments of weakness, when I was functioning on just two or three hours of sleep, exhausted from having given so much of myself both emotionally and physically, I reflected on my upbringing. I'd think back on how my parents had raised me and taught me to always find my inner strength and to persevere. I could still hear Dad's voice in my mind.

La vita è un combattimento. Life is a struggle that we must endure.

TWELVE

Teachable Moments

With each passing day, my son fell deeper into a world unknown to me.

"Giaci, Giaci, Giaci!" I called. He was two steps away but wouldn't even turn to look at me. He was enthralled in his Hot Wheels cars and the racetrack. I didn't think he knew what to do when his name was called. So, he did not respond, not even to turn to acknowledge me.

Each day, the distance between us grew. Each time I thought we were making progress, we became stuck in an endless loop, with Giaci running in his own world and me flailing in mine. The hope for connection flickered.

Christmas passed. I was seven months pregnant, and I was told by my obstetrician that most twins deliver early. The toilet training was not going that well, but one benefit of the kids and I all being together in the bathroom was that Giaci was not able to run away. I capitalized on this enforced closeness. I wanted us to master a reciprocal "I love you so much" outside of the wrestling game.

When he replied to "I love you so much" with his little "Love you so much, Mommy," that felt like enough for the day. Since he wasn't accomplishing his bathroom routine, I didn't feel like keeping either of us in that small space for long. We'd try again later.

"Who's ready for lunch?" I asked Lauren and Giaci. I held Giaci's hand and guided him to the kitchen, where I hoisted him up into his high chair. I had to make sure he was secure and belted in so he couldn't climb out and run into another room or hurt himself.

Lauren's hair bounced with each step she took. She asked me for a plate because she wanted a peanut butter and jelly sandwich.

I grabbed a few plastic plates but lost hold of them. They crashed onto the ceramic tile and scattered around me. The sound of the plates hitting the kitchen floor flipped a switch inside me, even though nothing was broken, and no one was hurt. I began to cry. I was exhausted, afraid, and uncomfortable in my body from all the changes happening to me physically. Giaci didn't even react, whereas Lauren leaned in toward me and touched my leg.

I couldn't even pick up the plates because of how pregnant I was. Bawling and panting for air, I just stared into space.

When I leaned back against the counter I couldn't even sit comfortably. I saw brown bouncy curls at my feet. Lauren was shuffling around, picking up the plates for me. When she noticed that my crying had eased, she looked up at me and said in her sweetest voice, "It's okay, Mommy, I can help you." With the pigtails on the sides of her head bouncing and her Muppet-like hands, she collected the plates and handed them to me, one at a time.

I continued to stare down at her. I had never lost it in front of my children like this before, but I was clearly having trouble holding in my emotions. I was stunned by Lauren's innocence and generosity toward me. Without knowing the pain and suffering I felt, she had known what to do, as usual.

Soon I'd have four children. Would the twins be independent like Lauren? Dependent like Giaci? Somewhere in between? Lauren's actions hit me harder than the plates hit the floor. My children needed me to toughen up and face our life.

Once Lauren was done cleaning, she took my hand and kissed it. That's when I realized that both of my hands were shaking. My fear wanted to be known; I had kept it sealed inside, but today it found a way to release itself in front of the kids. I couldn't let this happen. I wouldn't.

My little girl looked up at me with attentive eyes. I needed to be a good role model for her.

I wiped the tears away and bent down as far as I could to return her kiss. I made it to her forehead before wobbling back up. I wondered if I should talk to her about my outburst, but she was only three years old. How would I even begin to explain it? Instead, I stuffed the fear and pain so far down that it would take an excavator to dig it out, and I made her the sandwich she had been waiting for.

Lauren was in the observing phase of her development, which meant that my every move was being watched. It was a crucial time, and I wouldn't mess that up for her. As I made the sandwich, I watched her eyes follow me. Her mind was also two steps ahead of mine. When I grabbed the slices of bread, she glanced over to the cabinet where the jar of peanut butter was and then over to the object still labelled *fridge*, where the jelly lived. I placed all the items on the table and dragged a chair over so that my firstborn could have a better view of my every move.

It was a teachable moment, but I was the one being taught the lesson. As I demonstrated each step for Lauren, dividing the slices perfectly, spreading a little more peanut butter on her sandwich and a little more jam on Giaci's—just how they both liked it—I realized that I needed to break down and simplify each step for more effective learning. This was what *Giaci* needed!

A light went on in my mind: too many steps meant too much information for him. One little step at a time made more sense for his ability to acquire skills.

Lauren learned differently and had no problem acquiring a complex skill. From a young age, she had been able to pick up two, three, or four steps at a time. She naturally interacted with everyone she encountered without being prompted, as typically developing children did. Being social was instinctual for her. Her eyes didn't miss a thing, and her interest in others gave her the drive to implement her curiosity.

Giaci didn't learn in the same way. He had a short attention span and would lose interest quickly, often running off to something else that caught his eye. His learning had to be broken into small steps for it to make sense for him. He didn't process his environment like she did. He was unaware of his surroundings, and because he lived in his own world, he didn't know any different. He needed more guidance and more parameters for his learning.

My conversations with Lauren brightened my days. Not only did she entertain me, but she was also my biggest aide. She was always my little helper, wanting to please, participate, and provide support. Observing her constantly and noting the differences between her and her brother guided me on how to help Giaci learn.

* * *

Now that I had a new approach to teaching Giaci, I was more hopeful about his potty training, which turned into boot-camp drills. Every day, I'd pull Lauren into our march toward the bathroom, like soldiers parading joyfully down the hallway so that Giaci would follow our lead. In military style, we chanted, "Forward march, march, march!" We playfully stiffened our legs, swinging one arm six inches to the front and three inches to the rear. We then forged ahead into the bathroom, injecting fun into this repetitive act. Giaci chuckled as he watched and cautiously followed.

A regimented schedule guided our days and highlighted the importance of data collection. Every day for at least two weeks, I would record Giaci's exact liquid intake, the times he drank, and the times he went to the bathroom. A pattern soon emerged, so I incorporated placing him on the potty at strategic times. I also paired our march to the bathroom with saying the word *toilet*.

While he sat on the toilet, I would turn the faucet on in hopes of igniting the sensation. As soon as he did pee, we had the wildest "Pee

Party" celebration! These occurrences became more and more frequent, which solidified his learning and understanding.

Giaci now understood the difference between an "angry" face and a "happy" face, thanks to my vivid and consistent delivery of both. An angry face was paired with a deeper voice and a scowl, while a happy face was an energetic, illuminated expression accompanied by hugs, kisses, and tickles. He was clear on the difference and preferred the latter.

Every time he sat on the toilet at the scheduled time, I implemented the huge reinforcement. Seeing his delight motivated me even more. The notes I took clearly showed that we were making progress, but we were not quite there yet. The process was tedious and a lot of work, but it had to be followed. It was the only way.

As thrilled as I was by the possibility of him eventually being able to use the potty on his own, my head spun at the thought of how many other countless skills I would have to teach him.

My moments of peace were overwhelmed by a familiar anxiety. Although I desperately needed a moment of rest, looking down at my bursting belly, I knew I didn't have much time.

THIRTEEN

Play Date

When my old friend Antoniette called and asked me out for coffee, lunch, or a play date for our kids, I usually made excuses not to go. I didn't know how to be myself anymore or how to be social without breaking down. Being at home was safer; there, my emotions could burst and bubble to the surface with no one to see it. Out in the world, I was vulnerable.

But then one day when Antoinette called with an invitation, I said yes.

John said, "It'll be good for you! She's always been a good friend, and getting out may even be fun."

He always validated me before leaving for work, and he never left without giving the kids big hugs and kisses first. But still, John and I were tired, and our communication had started to fail. We never talked about the hard stuff, like how our lives had changed with Giaci's diagnosis; we just exchanged a few sweet words to get the other through the day. For a time, it broke my heart knowing that we'd drifted apart, especially with two babies on the way, but basic communication was all we could manage for now.

John was right about it being good to get out. It felt great to get out of the house, but also, I needed to get out of my own head, and Antoinette was just the friend for this. She had an easygoing personality and wasn't the type to cast judgment or question me or my son.

Back in high school, I had girlfriends who cared more about how they looked and the designer clothes they wore than the person they were. Antoinette wasn't like that. She didn't care what you wore or where you came from; what mattered to her was honesty and genuine friendship.

I knew it would be nice to reconnect with her. It had been almost three years since I'd seen her, and many months since I'd socialized with anyone other than my family.

When I told Lauren and Giaci that we were leaving the house for a play date, Lauren lit up. Giaci, seeing his sister's excitement, smiled as well, but he didn't fully comprehend what was going on. Spending most of our days inside, with few people coming by other than my parents and my in-laws, was weighing on Lauren the most. She would always ask me to go places, but I didn't have it in me.

"Mommy, can we go to the park?"

"Mommy, can we go for a walk?"

"Mommy, can we go to the corner store?"

I always responded with a "Not today, honey."

No matter how nervous I was about tackling a play date—without all our creature comforts and while making sure Giaci wouldn't run around for the entire visit—I had to do this for her and for myself.

I dressed Giaci and Lauren in play clothes, with both of them in summer shorts, T-shirts, and running shoes. They'd be ready to run around to their heart's content at the downtown community centre.

Before we left, I pulled Lauren aside. I had to make sure she wouldn't forget to be watchful of her brother. I knew she would be, but reiterating it made me feel a little better.

"Lauren, I'll hold Giaci as much as I can, but when you go into the play area, I won't be able to go with you. It's just for kids, so you have to make sure your brother is with you at all times because he doesn't know what to do."

She nodded and grabbed hold of her brother's arm as we got into the van. Giaci was oblivious to where we were going—he didn't comprehend my words or have the vocabulary, so he just followed Lauren's lead.

I gripped Giaci's hand as we entered the community centre, and Lauren walked freely beside us. We were greeted by the screeching voices of joyful and energetic children. I'd never seen my kids' faces light up so fast. Giaci reacted with a heightened excitement. He giggled happily, and his eyes widened as he scanned the entire play area. Visually and auditorily he was stimulated. He may not have understood my words in telling him where we were going, but to see and hear all the children running around, the bright colours, and sounds—this affected him. It was sensory overload for Giaci. His expression showed that he was processing all the information coming at him, and his hand vibrated in mine, wanting to wriggle out. There was a strong risk of him running off, which weighed heavily on me. I gripped him tighter. Without being able to move his captive hand, he flapped his other excitedly while his legs propelled him into continuous jumps. As we walked over to where Antoinette sat waving, Giaci was trying to calibrate to his new environment, launching himself into the air as he adjusted to all the stimuli.

To the left side of the industrial warehouse-sized room were nylon tunnels. These tubes had a steady stream of air pumping through them, causing them to inflate. They led to a bigger nylon-covered area where kids could play. Kids crawled inside the tunnels and manoeuvred their way into the covered tent-like play area. Giaci was giddy watching the other kids play. He laughed hysterically. He couldn't wait to join them. Lauren's attention was to the right, where there was a ball pit with an indoor playground and slides. Their outward displays of emotion were vastly different, and already my brain was in education-and-planning mode, trying to figure out which unique teaching steps I could apply to each of them on this fun afternoon.

"Rita! Over here!" Antoinette called out as we got closer. She was near the tunnels, and even from that distance, her voice rang out clear over the sound of children at play. Being a mom meant developing the amplified voice of a sports announcer.

My response was softer, and I tried to push away the exhaustion that was slipping through in the squeak of my voice. "Wow! This place is amazing." I looked around and then bent down to meet her son Michael's eyes. "And your little man is getting so big already!"

"Don't remind me! Time is flying. Look at Lauren and Giaci!"

"He's ready to run," I said, sounding deflated even to my own ears. "I don't think I can hold him back anymore."

"Don't! This is the perfect place to let him loose. We'll watch him together," she responded. It sounded so easy coming from her. *Just let him loose*—my absolute worst fear.

I pressed my lips together, trying to hide the sweat already forming above my upper lip, and bent down to talk to Lauren. "Sweetie, let's start at the tunnels, okay? Can you stay with your brother?"

She met my eyes, and it was clear she understood. A moment later, she turned to her brother and said, "Come on, Giaci! You want to go in the tunnel?" Lauren grabbed his hand and pulled him.

When they started to run, my heart did too, but I had to try to let the anxiety go, if only for my sanity.

Antoinette and I stood nearby, keeping our eyes on the kids as we chatted. Lauren was showing Giaci how to get into the tunnel, but he just watched her go inside the tube, his eyes wide. He then peeked into the tube with his round, brush-cut head. He didn't follow but kept eyeing the inside, laughing like a banshee. His eyes flew back and forth between the tube and me. While Lauren and Michael were both already deep in the centre of the tunnels, Giaci continued to peer in, taking pleasure in the sensory stimulation: the air blowing on his face, the smells in the tunnel, the lighting changes, and whatever else was sparking his brain.

"Do you think he'll go in?" Antoinette turned to me and laughed. "I can't take the anticipation! He seems to want to."

"I think he might need a little help," I said, making my way over to Giaci. I braced my belly and got down on my knees to crawl over to him. When he noticed me, his expression exploded with joy. His exultation thrilled me. He leaned down to inspect the tube again and show it to me, exposing his little butt in the air. I gave him a big shove that catapulted him into the tube; I had to do this or else he would have stayed there the whole time, unable to take the next step on his own. I could hear Antoinette laughing from our spot while I watched Giaci's little shadow explore the tunnel. He laughed the whole way. Once he was in, I relaxed a little, knowing he was somewhat contained.

"Okay," I said as I walked back over to Antoinette, brushing my hands together to signal that the job was done. "So, what's new with you, Ant?" I asked. I had almost forgotten what adult conversation felt like.

"Nothing much, just busy with the family and teaching."

We jumped into teacher talk, keeping our conversation surface-level with chatter about our school assignments. Antoinette and I went to the faculty of education together, so our work came up often. Soon enough, we were back to reminiscing about the olden days, back in high school.

"Remember the hair we had? The bigger the better!" I said as we chuckled, recalling the gallons of hairspray we used to keep our back-combed hair up.

"What about when we went to France?" In our last year of university, Antoinette and I did an exchange program, attending classes at the University of Nice in France. After classes we would walk from our dorm, which was on top of a picturesque mountainside, down the rocky trail until we could smell the delicious aromas of the pastries and croissants coming from the bakery in the *Vieille Ville*, the old town. We baked in the southern sun of the French Riviera on the pebbled beaches, enjoying our vibrant, carefree early twenties. The memories were heavenly.

"Oh, I could go for a plate of pasta Bolognese at that restaurant we used to go to on the beach," I said, my mouth watering just thinking about it. "Those were the days, eh?"

Antoinette nodded in agreement.

"My favourite was people-watching at the café while we ate ice cream," I added.

We giggled like schoolgirls.

"It was awesome—school, the beach, then dancing at the disco." Antoinette nodded as she spoke, almost in disbelief that we had shared such a magical time.

That life seemed so different from what I was living now. Back then, all I had to worry about was myself.

With Antoinette, I felt myself ease back into the person I had once been and began releasing my rigid, self-imposed restrictions. I didn't turn this playtime into a teachable moment. I didn't break down steps. I just *was*. It was almost uncomfortable to be this carefree, delightful person now, to laugh and talk about events that had seemed so weighty in school but now felt feathery light compared to my current life.

"Things have changed so much, haven't they?" I asked.

"I guess that's life, isn't it?"

We continued to talk, each with one eye on the kids.

Antoinette was a breezy friend, never asking anything too serious, which was exactly what my brain needed at this point in my life. All thoughts of the future, of the twins, of Giaci faded into the background—still there, just dulled.

Motherhood never came with a break, but it was nice to pretend even if just for a minute that I wasn't *Mommy* or *teacher*, just *Rita*. I tried to relish every second before we had to go back home, not knowing when the next such break would come.

When we got home, the kids were exhausted and fell asleep almost immediately. While they slept, I just stood by their bedroom door and thought about this beautiful day that I'd had to myself. I never wanted it to end.

FOURTEEN

Twin Sisters

The phone rang early in the morning. "Hello?" I answered.

"Hi Ri," my mom said.

"Hi Ma."

"What's wrong?" she asked.

"No, nothing," I answered.

"You okay? The kids?"

"Yes, we are good, thanks."

Each morning, it took all the energy I could muster to put on an Oscar-winning performance. I chose to conceal my fears; I didn't dare discuss Giaci's diagnosis. Instead, I pulled at my hair and tried to pretend that it was all just a bad dream. I did what I thought strong mothers should do: I hid as much as I could to spare the grandparents the heartache and worry.

Whenever my voice sounded tired, I attributed it to the pregnancy. *Tutto va bene ma sono stanca*, I'd explain in Italian, adding that the babies were keeping me up, rather than placing the blame on Giaci.

Again and again I wondered, *How can I tell them about all the delays their grandson is experiencing?*

When the words tried to bubble up, I always forced them back down. A diagnosis of autism hadn't existed in their time, or if it did, they never spoke of it. How would I explain it to them?

* * *

The twins were coming.

As the contractions seemed to get closer and stronger, I began running around the house grabbing the bags I had prepared. One bag was for Giaci; he was going to Nonna Maria's. Another was for Lauren; she was going to Nonna Carolina's. The third was mine for the hospital. As I tried to subdue the bursts of pain with deep-breathing techniques, I called John to let him know it was time. He rushed home to get us.

When we got to the hospital, the doctor told us that these were false contractions, causing me a mix of sadness and relief. I wanted to meet my two new babies, but I didn't feel ready. I felt even less prepared than I had before Lauren was born. There was still much to do and much to teach Giaci. Would I ever be ready?

For an entire month, John and I would rush over to the hospital just to be sent home. It was like when Giaci would watch a movie on videotape. He would stop and rewind, stop and rewind, over and over again. To him, familiarity was comforting.

Life—and now these contractions—seemed to be happening in the same way.

I was terrified at the thought of the twins being negatively affected by the on-again, off-again contractions. Once again everything felt out of my control, leaving me helpless. I was almost used to the feeling. Even the way the twins were about to enter the world wasn't how I expected it to be.

Five weeks before my due date, the doctor was confident that the twins were big and healthy enough to be delivered. He estimated their weight to be about six pounds each and was satisfied that we could prepare for their delivery. The constant contractions and strain on my body were taking its toll, but my emotional turmoil was far worse. No one knew the struggles we faced in our home.

What if they are autistic too? I wondered. *What will I do?*

I couldn't let my mind go there—but I did.

It was the day after Valentine's Day, and when we got to the hospital, the doctor told us that this time we were not going to be sent home. The nurses quickly prepared me for surgery. These babies were coming, and John and I would just have to persevere. It was what we were good at.

"Are you all right, honey?" the nurse asked while wheeling me away to check my vitals.

I was so in my own head that I didn't know how to answer. I mouthed *Yes*, but no sound came out. She nodded back, passing it off as new-mother syndrome. This was an entirely different and paralyzing fear, though.

Is John this nervous too? I looked around for him.

When I spotted him, his face looked the exact opposite of mine, as usual. His expression was open and bright, excited for the twins' arrival. Part of me was envious. I wished that I could enjoy the same anticipation; instead, the joy was clogged by other badgering thoughts.

John and I had the same circular conversation almost every night. It would begin with me asking what he would do if the twins were like Giaci.

He would then act like there was nothing wrong. "We'll work through it," he always said. "We've come this far, and we'll keep going." His face was always smooth when he said this.

All the worry lines had jumped from his face onto mine. It was frustrating.

Now I kept staring at him, wondering if he would flinch with fear, or if he would show any emotion other than complete, measured calm. When he didn't, I tried to absorb his ease, to breathe it in as if it were a vapour emanating from his pores.

John's sister Josie stepped in front of me between breaths.

"How are you doing, Ri?" she asked.

She was my plus-one in the delivery room alongside John. Josie was a neonatal intensive care unit nurse, which could be helpful during the delivery—a planned C-section. She would also be there as extra support for John in case he needed it.

Weeks before the delivery I had spoken to Josie about joining us. "You know how your brother is at the sight of blood," I said. "He's never seen a surgery, so please keep an eye on him. He may faint. Even though he turned out the biggest in your family, he's also the softest."

"Don't worry. If he faints, I'll just push him aside and tend to the babies," she said, and we chuckled. John and Josie had always shared a loving sibling banter.

When it was time for them to do the incision, they draped a curtain across my shoulders.

"Jos…" I grabbed my sister-in-law's hand firmer than intended. "Please be my eyes, will you? You'll tell me…"

"I'll tell you everything. You'll be fine." She tapped my hand, as if politely telling me to loosen its viselike grip before walking to the other side of the curtain. She stood in the middle, half of her on my side and half on John's to support us both.

Anticipation and excitement filled the sterile air as the doctor began to cut. It was an eerie sensation to feel the tugging and manipulation, but no physical pain.

Josie gave me words to listen to—not quite like a sports announcer giving a running commentary of the game, like I'd hoped. At least I was able to visualize it in my head.

Meanwhile, I was fixated on John, who was deep in thought, with furrowed eyebrows hiding his hazel eyes. His eyebrows kept going up and down with the surgeon's every movement. Then they bolted straight up when the doctor pulled the first twin out.

I waited to hear a cry, and when it seemed like too much time was passing in silence, I asked what was taking so long.

It was ghastly silent.

I could see that everyone was watching the miracle of life happening.

But I needed to hear my new baby cry! Why wasn't she crying? Did someone or something take her voice? I began to shake.

"Someone answer me!" I shrieked.

Josie was just about to respond when the sound came. The baby cried. It was a beautiful girl. A tear trickled down my face, but it wasn't over. I needed to hear the other one. I trembled with uneasiness as everyone's attention went back to the other side of the curtain. I felt removed from the process, while everyone stood and watched me give birth.

Since I could not see what was going on, I relied on my other senses. I focused on the sterile smell, my dry mouth, the doctor's hands tugging and pulling at my abdomen as he guided my babies out of my womb. Sounds were magnified. The nurses clanked the scalpels and clamps together before handing them over to the doctor. Their feet slid around the room with minimal sound.

John and Josie were still, all breath and no movement.

I sighed, waiting for a second cry.

"Please, God, hurry," I whispered to myself. "I don't think I can take this anymore."

Then it happened. A second strong cry.

"Oh God, please make sure they're all right," I pleaded, trying to make a deal with my Superior Being.

Another tear rolled off my face, but this time Josie saw it. She wiped it gently off my face with her medical glove and smiled at me for a second, not wanting to take her eyes off the miraculous moment of her nieces being born.

Carolina and Maria Rosa had arrived—my adorable, angelic, identical twin daughters. I released an enormous sigh of relief that the twins were physically strong enough not to need a ventilator or medical support of any kind. They were almost six pounds each, and their rosy, pink complexions were sublime.

Still, the unknown of the twins' cognitive well-being occupied my thoughts. I couldn't fully enjoy the beauty of having created two new lives because of the fear that *their* bright futures might be stolen, too.

Before I could hold the girls, and before the doctor put me back together, there was one more procedure that needed to be done.

"Prepare for tubal ligation," the doctor said to the nurses around him.

The nurses obeyed his request, and I heard them shuffling back to life. The doctor then peeked over the curtain to speak to me. "We're tying your tubes now. You're sure?"

I nodded. I had signed all the necessary consent forms before coming to the hospital. It was set. As I lay there helplessly open—physically and emotionally—I searched the room for John. This was a decision we had made together prior to coming to the hospital. We agreed not to have any more children, and to enforce this, a tubal ligation made sense. Four children were enough for us.

But now, as the doctor asked me if I was sure, confusion swept over me. I suddenly wasn't sure that either of us had thought this through. I needed John's calm nature to reassure me. I hoped he would jump in with logic, guidance, and reassurance.

"John. Only one boy! You'll have only one boy." My stuttering voice revealed my inner panic, as if this were the pivotal importance of my reproductive ability. I wasn't the one who determined the sex of our children, yet I felt responsible that one boy wasn't enough. That *our boy* wouldn't be enough. Our cultural ideology was always present within me, that Italian belief—like the belief of many other cultures—that sons were of primary importance. For Italian men, having boys was important for carrying on the paternal name. At an Italian wedding, the traditional toast given to a bride and groom is to wish them many male offspring.

Tanti figli maschi! the guests would shout. *Many sons.*

As I lay on the operating table, I thought about how Giaci was not a typically developing boy; my husband was not getting the same father/son experience as other fathers do. A cultural obligation suddenly came over me, a belief defined by self-denial. I knew that I shouldn't have more children—I already struggled with caring for the ones I had—but I was willing to define myself as *sacrificata*, sacrificing myself to meet my husband's wishes.

My mind continued to race as I waited for direction from John, as did the doctor and nurses. The room stood frozen in time as we all shifted our eyes to John.

Then he spoke:

"Rita, one boy is all I want. We have a beautiful family."

His affirmation melted my heart. That was enough. As he finished speaking, the nurse brought twin A, cocooned in a pink blanket, to him. Twin B was handed to Josie. Still lying on the operating table, I couldn't stop staring. John stared at one baby and then the other, beaming with pride.

"They are exactly the same," he said.

And with four children, our family was complete.

FIFTEEN

"Holy Crap, Lauren!"

Compared to Lauren and Giaci, the twins were tiny. I could fit them both into one crib, and that's what I often did since they settled better when they were closer together, probably because they'd been in such close quarters for so long. When they slept, I enjoyed the moments of stillness. Carolina was always reaching out to hold Maria Rosa's hand or vice versa. I loved it!

After my morning routine with Giaci and Lauren, we'd all tiptoe past the babies' room to go into the kitchen for breakfast. I'd plop Giaci into his highchair and strap him in, while Lauren sat in her booster seat manoeuvring her chubby little hands to secure her own seatbelt.

"I want Cheerios, Mommy," she said one day, staring at the cereal box. "I think Giaci wants them too." She looked over at him like she was his spokesperson. His wide-eyed smile didn't look any different to me, but Lauren spoke for him, and she had started to decide what he needed and wanted. She just took it upon herself to make decisions for him. They were both able to feed themselves, so I took the opportunity to pour myself a bowl to eat alongside them.

Once we were finished, I left the dirty dishes on the table and walked the children to the bathroom to brush their teeth. Giaci needed help. Covering his little hand with mine, I guided the toothbrush in small circles around each of his tiny teeth as he squirmed, sitting on the counter by the bathroom sink.

As I stood there focusing on Giaci's teeth, Lauren brushed her own, standing tall on her pink step stool. Even with a brush lodged in her mouth, she had much to say. She was a born conversationalist.

"Giaci, stop moving so much! Mommy needs to clean your teeth. You don't want your teeth to fall out, do you? You won't look good without teeth, and then how will you ever be able to eat Nonna's bread?" She went on and on like this without taking a breath or spitting out the toothpaste that seeped out of her mouth. Then she glanced over at me and nodded, as if to acknowledge our co-leadership in this small army. I chuckled.

The twins were good daytime sleepers, and since they still weren't up after our bathroom adventure, I decided to put Giaci in his highchair so I could clean up the breakfast mess. I asked Lauren to fetch her favourite book and gave Giaci a See 'n Say toy to keep him busy. The repetitive movement of this toy was exactly what he liked.

"The cow says 'moo!'" the toy repeated over and over again, and each time Giaci would giggle and slam his hands on the table as if to say "Again!" He didn't repeat the phrase the toy intoned. Instead, his eyes fixated on the movement of the arrow. This was an enjoyable preoccupation for him.

Normally, Lauren would bring her books to the kitchen so we could read them together and try to engage her brother, but this morning, after several minutes, she still hadn't returned. I didn't want to call after her, for fear of waking the babies, so once I finished washing the dishes, I whisper-called for her.

"I'm in here, Mommy, with the twins. I take care of them for you." Her voice carried from the babies' room.

My face crinkled. Knowing that Giaci was secure in his chair and entertained by animal sounds, I went to the twins' room to find Lauren.

I opened the door to find Lauren sitting in the crib with the twins. My heart froze in fear as I envisioned her climbing up the crib bars with her pint-sized legs and falling into the crib where the twins lay peacefully sleeping.

"Holy crap, Lauren!" The words slipped out. I couldn't stop picturing her slipping and landing on the twins. She could have squished them!

She just sat there, cross-legged and wedged into the corner of the crib, with a sweet, naive look on her face. She smiled down at the twins and kept a watchful eye on them.

"Lauren…" I scowled, trying to contain my volume, since apparently their big sister climbing into their crib hadn't woken the babies.

With a blank look on her face, Lauren turned toward me. She was unsure of what she had done wrong. How could I scold her caring intentions? I scooped her up, and she wrapped her spunky arms around my neck as we tiptoed out of the nursery.

"Lauren, Mommy doesn't want to see you climb into the crib like that again, okay, honey? I know you love your baby sisters and want to help Mommy, but you can't go into the crib, okay?"

"Okay, Mommy," Lauren answered as I put her down in the kitchen. She ran off to fetch her favourite book, having already forgotten how she had frightened me. Disaster averted—for now.

PART TWO

At the Threshold

SIXTEEN

ABA Is Evidence-Based Therapy

It was the end of the summer of 1999. The twins were now eighteen months old, Giaci was almost four, and Lauren was five and a half. I had been a mother of four for more than a year, but I was still adjusting to motherhood.

John worked harder than any other man I knew. He would hurry from his busy full-time job to his second job of back-breaking construction labour. When he came home for dinner each day, I could see the physical toll our life was taking on him. Some days I'd just pack an extra meal for him, and he'd skip the dinnertime visit altogether. I only caught glimpses of his work life: a farmer's tan around his arms, calloused hands reaching for his construction clothes, and sore joints snapping as he bent down to kiss the kids.

These were the fragments of our life together.

I wondered what John thought of me when he came home. Maybe he saw my bruised, battered arms from having to carry the twins and Giaci around. Or the dishevelled hair and the unmanicured nails that were bitten from the anxiety that gnawed at me. Or my drooping eyes from endless exhaustion. The only thing he couldn't see was inside my mind; no matter how beaten my body may have looked, my mind was worse off. I was locked in negativity and depression.

I spent most days going head-to-head with Giaci, trying to decipher what he was thinking and how to best communicate with him.

Working on basic skills with Giaci was becoming harder to squeeze into my daily schedule. I was back to teaching elementary students part-time, but I was still a full-time mother. Once I was finished with my students, I would load up the kids in the van at the daycare, pick up the twins from one or the other nonna's house, and go home. Between cooking and home maintenance, the work never stopped. On top of that there was the new addition of extracurricular lessons and practice time for things like piano, dance, and gymnastics for Lauren, swimming lessons, appointments with the speech pathologist and sensory integration therapist for Giaci. The speech pathologist worked on getting more language out of Giaci. The therapist applied sensory integration techniques such as deep pressure, brushing, a weighted vest, and swinging to help calm his anxious body. These professionals also gave me homework. The brushing and weighted vest had to be applied for a specific amount of time, twice a day, and that time varied depending on his progress.

Giaci's special education teacher at daycare gave me a laundry list of goals she was working on with him each week so we could continue to implement these at home. This week, we had to practise circle time at home and get Giaci to sit and participate. To do this, I had the twins join us as two more participants. Lauren, Giaci, Carolina, Maria, and I held hands, walking in a circle on the carpet in the living room, smiling and giggling as we sang "Ring Around the Rosie." By the time we got to "We all fall down," Giaci was singing a few words and falling to the ground along with us. It was fun for all of us. This activity was to encourage language—and it was working. Circle time, movement activities, imitation games, pretend play and encouraging language and social interaction would take up all my spare time, which was already scarce.

When the kids were in bed that night and John was still at his second job, I scoured the internet for anything that could help us help Giaci.

My eyes had flickered across the phrase *applied behavioural analysis*

(ABA) multiple times, and the more I read about it, the more I thought that this was what I wanted and needed for Giaci. ABA is an evidence-based therapy, I read, that could improve social communication and learning skills through positive reinforcement. ABA treatment is useful in teaching behaviours to children with autism who may otherwise not pick up these behaviours on their own, as other children might. The intervention consists of breaking down skills into their simplest components, rewarding children positively, and then generalizing the skills into a natural environment. ABA therapy is based on the finding that when behaviour is rewarded, it is more likely to be repeated.

I had already seen this type of learning system succeed with Giaci, like when we were able to induce him to say, "I love you," with the reward of wrestling with John. Giaci clearly responded to this approach, but I needed to know more before fully diving in.

Applied Behavior Analysis (ABA) Therapy was first developed in the 1970s by psychologists Ivar Lovaas and Robert Koegel at UCLA, I read. I skimmed ahead and picked out the parts that stood out to me, such as *increased improvement in children's IQ scores* and *an increase in functional learning.*

Yet all these results were produced in children who received forty hours per week of ABA therapy. How could we possibly get Giaci to engage for that long? What would it cost us?

More importantly, what I read indicated that starting at a young age resulted in the best outcome. Early intervention is fundamental. For young children with autism, this means that the skills needed to reach their full potential are taught early, when brain plasticity is much more pronounced, and the impact of intervention is much more comprehensive.

By providing intervention early on, I knew we could mitigate the severity of the behaviours that Giaci struggled with most and perhaps alter the trajectory of his development. The brain is malleable, after all, meaning that we are constantly learning depending on experiences and exposure.

Could that happen for Giaci? The thought of it brought me to tears. As I continued reading, my eyes were opened to the mixed views on ABA. Many felt that ABA was a source of trauma, forcing autistic people to mask stims and act "less autistic." In fact, many people view ABA as child abuse, forcing a child to do what someone else wants them to do. This was astonishing to me. I didn't want to hurt my son. I wouldn't hurt him. But I did have to give this intervention a try. After all, intervention approaches are effective in compliance with reinforcements. This was the philosophy I followed as an educator.

I started looking at programs available in our area and found that the government of Ontario had begun a program offering behavioural services to children with autism, but only until the age of six. Thankfully, Giaci was nearly four now, so he still met their criteria, but there was an endless waitlist for their services.

Being on this waitlist was torturous. I refused to be another number. I called the program offices constantly, hoping there was an opening. Each time I called, I heard vague, empty voices on the other end of the line telling me to be patient or that they had no new information for me. Those words made my cheeks burn with anger.

I became relentless in placing these calls. I began forcing myself onto the phone every single day. By the fourth day in a row, they knew who I was.

"Yes, this is Rita from Windsor again," I said, almost annoying myself with the tone I used.

"I'm sorry, but there hasn't been any change in the waitlist since we spoke yesterday," said the female voice who answered robotically, as if her response were scripted.

"Okay, I'll try back again tomorrow," I said. I wanted her to know who I was.

My purpose was clear.

Each day that we were on the waitlist was another day lost without one-on-one attention. There was no way I could perform the techniques on my own; I didn't have a clue of where or how to start. I couldn't sit in my helplessness anymore, so I charged forward every day.

I also didn't hide my frustration with the service provider, letting every emotion I'd been holding in for so long spill out.

And one day, I said, "This is the only intervention available to my son, and we have to wait?" My voice rose. "You're telling me that if my son had cancer, a doctor would tell us that we have to wait our turn for treatment? No, I don't think so. Help would be offered immediately! But with this developmental disorder, we have to wait? I'm sure you know that early intervention is crucial." I paused, hoping my words would finally have an impact. "Surely you can help us!" I didn't leave it an open-ended question. My voice was forceful, and I used the fear, anger, and helplessness I had accumulated over the years to propel me forward. On the outside, I spoke with conviction, but inside, I was scared, shaking.

Unfortunately, this rant got me nowhere. It was like being in a glass bubble. My face was mashed up against the glass, my shouts unheard.

Despite this and other tirades that flowed from my feelings of abandonment, the strangers on the other end of the phone never seemed fazed by me or my pleas. My words were nothing new to them; countless parents were probably giving them the same spiel every ten minutes. We had to become the voice for our children who were being impacted. If we didn't speak up, who would?

A part of me didn't care what these strangers thought of me, but another part was still worried that they thought I was out of my mind. I was still deeply rooted in my people-pleasing ways. I didn't want to offend anyone or hurt their feelings. My parents had always provided me with a safe haven, raising me to be compassionate and empathetic toward others. Even now, when I think back on the days and days of borderline rude and aggressive calls, I recoil. That wasn't me. I derived joy from pleasing others. I craved approval from others. An endless yearning for approval circulated in my veins like the blood that filled them.

One day back in seventh grade, I'd worn my favourite outfit to school. It was a frilly white blouse with a dainty bow at the neck, red gaucho pants that flowed ever so softly, and a red-buttoned sleeveless vest. When I arrived at school that morning, excited to show off my outfit, I took off my coat and I noticed Krista looking me over. I stood up straight, shoulders back and chin up, so she could better admire my clothes.

But her expression changed. Her eyebrows dropped and her face crinkled as she said, "What are you wearing? That is so ugly!"

I turned multiple shades of red and couldn't muster a comeback. With drooped shoulders, I slouched as if I were a balloon someone had taken a pin to, exploding and then deflating completely.

As I walked away, Krista added, "You look ridiculous, Rita!"

At lunch, I ran all the way home and changed into a more "Krista-approved" outfit.

Back then, I should have realized that *my* opinion mattered more. I loved that outfit and had worn it with pride.

I tried to remember that now, with these voices on the other end of the line. Every time I called, I tried not to imagine them thinking, *Oh, there's that bitchy mom again. What does she think she's accomplishing?* My personal beliefs and obedient cultural upbringing pushed me to back down, to give in, but my maternal duty was stronger, and it held me in place. My son's future depended on it. The goal was to increase his IQ scores and increase functional learning. The fear of not getting this intervention that could help us attain our goal immediately ignited the advocate in me.

And so, every day, I placed my routine phone calls, and every day, my efforts seemed to fall on deaf ears. I couldn't stand the wait anymore; it was emotionally exhausting.

"We have to go private," I said to John one day, exhausted by another failed call. "I found a few good leads, but they're expensive." I let the words hang between us. The average cost of ABA was $40,000 to $60,000.

I was about to ramble, still fired up from another futile call, to try to convince John that ABA therapy was the only way, when he broke through my thoughts.

"I know you've been working hard with him, Ri. He needs this and so do you. We'll try it and make it work," he said as he gently brushed my shoulder on his way out.

We'll make it work. Those were our magic words. We were always trying to make it work. Now, there was no other way. We would have to make it work.

* * *

For a month I held interviews for a private therapist and finally landed on a vibrant young therapist, Shipu.

Shipu was not the cheapest therapist we interviewed, but she came highly recommended and had experience in the ABA field. Her bright eyes and long, straight black hair commanded the room—so much so that even Giaci noticed her.

Our first meeting was informal. I asked Shipu to sit at the kitchen table so I could go over her resumé and ask her a few questions. While we spoke, my four children sat on the couch in the living room nearby. The twins were almost two years old. I had put on a *Scooby Doo* video to keep them occupied. As usual, Giaci ran back and forth and back and forth the whole time, flapping his hands. He couldn't sit still for long, not even for an entire video. The girls were accustomed to this behaviour, so they didn't react at all, but I could see Shipu's gaze shift respectfully from me to Giaci and back.

When we had finished our conversation, she rose to her feet and walked past the living room toward the front door. Before reaching it, she stopped right in the middle of Giaci's running path. She stood there motionless, expressionless, and silent, blocking his way. He stopped, took stock of her, and then continued running from where he had left off. To many, it may not have seemed like an interaction, but to me it did. At that moment, Shipu had been noticed by my son, who typically didn't stop for anyone.

That evening, after talking it over with John, I called Shipu.

"Shipu, we would like to hire you to work with our son. Are you interested?"

"Of course," she said. She accepted without hesitation and immediately began asking me several questions.

"What does Giaci like?" she asked with much interest.

"He loves chips and jumping on the single-person indoor mini trampoline that we have downstairs," I answered almost proudly. "He also likes high fives and praise."

"What would you like to see him learn?" she asked. I could hear faint jotting in the background.

There was a long list of potential answers to this loaded question. I stared into space until my vision blurred, pondering how best to answer.

"There are so many things that he *needs* to learn," I answered with a vulnerability in my voice. "But I would just love to hear him tell me about his day." My throat swelled but I choked the emotion down. Shipu was really listening, and her pencil never left the page. I could hear the scratching sound of graphite and my every word being scribbled on the other end.

My responses seemed to flow more after that emotional release.

"I want him to answer simple questions like what his name is. I want him to be able to put on his own clothes and shoes." I went on, listing both the essentials and the wishes. I took a quick breath, waiting for her to stop me, but she didn't. "And I'd like to see his eye contact increase." I finished with, "Whatever you think he needs to learn is what I want. I just want to see him learning as much as possible."

Shipu continued to write frantically for a few minutes, and then she explained her process. She would record data on every task analysis, also known as a lesson. Apparently, a task analysis is the process of breaking a skill down into smaller, more manageable components. Once a task analysis is complete, it can be used to teach learners a skill that is too challenging to teach all at once. As an educator, I understood this.

"I will need two chairs, a table, pencils, paper, chips in a bowl…" She listed off the items she would need when she would come to our house to work with him. It made sense to have them ready for her, so she didn't have to bring materials back and forth. "I need you to photocopy the papers that I'll bring, and I will also give you a list of small toys that you need to have ready for me."

Shipu paused as if waiting for a response. When she realized that none was forthcoming, she continued.

"We'll discuss his progress in regular meetings so you're aware of what we're working on and how to implement this learning when I'm not there."

When she paused again, I burst out, "Absolutely! Thank you so much!" Gratitude poured out of me through the phone.

Shipu, like the government strangers on the phone, was unfazed by my devotion. She'd probably seen it dozens of times before, but this was a first for us; she was the first person who could help get our son to socialize and communicate with others. I had to believe it would work.

A hunger rumbled inside of me to start this intensive therapy immediately. I'd had a taste of success, and I now craved more. There was still a sense of vulnerability, though, because we were not in control. We were at Shipu's mercy, and she was in the driver's seat. All I could do was trust that she would help him increase independence, grow his language skills and equip him to pursue a prosperous life—a life everyone would be proud of.

I imagined my parents gloating about their star grandson the way they once praised me and my brothers.

"My daughter is on the honour roll," Dad would boast. "She is a very good student." He even occasionally handed me a five-dollar bill as a reward for my accomplishments.

I knew they hoped Giaci would achieve similar academic success and eventually go off to college or university. In my father's eyes, that was the only way to succeed.

John and I would be proud of Giaci no matter what, but deep down I still craved that type of acceptance from others. If they knew that Giaci had cognitive impairments and was intellectually delayed, would they accept our son? How would they treat him?

My fear of others judging my son was paralyzing, and it kept me from opening up to others. I couldn't control what anyone else thought or said. All I could control was how I responded to them.

SEVENTEEN

Let's Get to Work

The next day, Shipu arrived promptly, ready to begin. We gave her all the support we could to allow her to perform her magic. I had all the educational materials, writing supplies, and small toys she had requested, plus a little bowl of plain potato chips. I desperately hoped that somewhere, between these small items, we might find answers. I set everything up in the living room downstairs so they would not be interrupted.

Giaci had no idea what was about to happen, but to be honest, neither did I. I didn't know if they would play, or if she would navigate through lessons the way I'd done. If nothing else, Shipu wouldn't have three additional children at her side. While she worked with Giaci in the afternoon, I was able to get chores done around the house and made sure my other children got individual attention from me.

When Shipu entered the house, Giaci was immediately mesmerized by her. I'd never seen him like this with anyone else. His eyes stayed on her for more than a minute—a record amount of time. In retrospect, I realize her aura was calm and confident and she was an unfamiliar face.

"Come on, Giaci. Let's get to work." Shipu guided his hand up to hers as they calmly made their way downstairs.

There was no hesitation on his end, which made the girls feel like there was something to be experienced in the basement.

"We want to go too, Mommy!" Lauren spoke for her siblings as usual.

"No, honey, this is for Giaci only," I answered, hoping she would accept that.

Maria and Carolina, now three years old, didn't fully hear the entire conversation, but their eyes seemed to glisten at the idea of moving from their spot. They all wanted to join in on the activities, but I had to stop and distract them with something else.

"Okay, girls, let's read a book together. Who wants to choose a really good book?"

Maria quickly grabbed her favourite book, and we settled down to read her selection. I tried my best to keep them entertained, animating my words to keep their attention.

At first, we couldn't hear what was happening below, but soon our activity was interrupted by Shipu's repetitive words.

"Sit down, Giaci," her firm voice echoed through the floor. "Sit down."

I tried to remain focused on the girls. This was *our* time, after all. But it was also Giaci's first session with Shipu, and one of my ears would perk up at each of Shipu's commands. Even worse, I wanted so badly to be down there with them that my imagination was beginning to fill in the blanks of what could be happening between the two of them. Was he was doing everything she asked him to do? Perhaps he was smiling and responding?

As I listened in on Shipu arranging the items on the little table, I pictured her physically guiding Giaci to sit on his chair. I'd been in that position many times myself and knew this was no easy task. She'd have to physically manoeuvre him to where he had to go. With me—but only with me—a single look could prompt him to follow my directions. Part of me wanted to run downstairs to make it happen, but I couldn't. I had to stay upstairs.

"Look at me, Giaci," Shipu said in a deepened voice. She had likely finally gotten him to sit. "Giaci," she kept repeating in the same tone, to get his attention. Over and over, she would repeat his name, just like my brain was doing. I kept imagining Giaci stuck in this therapy for hours.

Eventually, Lauren snapped me out of it.

"Mommy, we want to play."

"I'm sorry, honey. Okay, what do you girls want to play?" I said, trying to refocus myself.

Carolina went to get her violin. "Concert time," she said. Maria perked up at the idea and didn't hesitate to get hers as well.

"I'll be the conductor," Lauren said as she picked up her baton.

"Mommy, you listen," Maria said.

Once the squeaking toy violins started, it was harder to keep one ear on them and one on their brother. My mind was neither here nor there.

Shipu was still a stranger, after all. It seemed perfectly normal to go check on her. I selected a small task that would take me downstairs and allow me to break the barrier between me and my son. I needed to see how he was doing. Was he already better? Was he in agony? Did he know that it was all my fault? Could he sense that I was trying to help him?

"Girls, you keep playing. I'll be right back," I said.

Laundry was my chosen task, since the laundry room was downstairs near the therapy area. As I picked random clothing items from around the kids' rooms to fill my basket, I thought about how I would tiptoe past Shipu and Giaci. My desire to know what was happening was intense.

As I walked by the session-in-progress, I saw Shipu pointing at objects on the table. When she was done, she said, "Show me book." When he pointed, she positively reinforced his efforts with, "Good boy. Nice job!" Her words were paired with a positive smile, to show Giaci that this was the response or behaviour she wanted to see.

After a few minutes of this task, she made a new request.

"Do this," she said as she jumped up, waiting for him to imitate her action. She was relentless in her delivery and didn't seem fazed by the slow progress. After many blank-faced moments, he jumped up and down, but he looked exhausted by her countless requests and directions.

I stood there for several minutes watching, laundry basket in hand. Only when Giaci noticed me did I flip around the corner and bolt upstairs, realizing that I'd left the girls to fend for themselves.

When I got back upstairs, the girls were wide-eyed and wondering what it was like in the "special room" downstairs. Lauren in particular was curious.

"How's Giaci, Mommy? What's he doing? Is he having fun?"

The twins stared at me through their round glasses, waiting for my answer. I didn't have the heart to tell Lauren—or myself—that I didn't think Giaci was having fun at all, especially because I didn't hear any giggling. All I heard was repetitive demands from Shipu. It didn't sound like fun to me.

"This is really good for Giaci, girls." It was all I could say, and I wasn't even sure it was true.

As Shipu's visits increased, Giaci became more distressed. He would see her coming through the window and begin flapping his arms. He'd even run away and hide, refusing to go downstairs with her. I didn't know what else to do except walk him down myself to the therapy area.

"Come on, honey, let's go downstairs with Shipu. It's time to get to work," I said as calmly as I could. "No," he replied as he tried to free himself from my grip. I felt a sting of desperation behind my tears, and guilt twisted my stomach, but we had to try.

The first few sessions involved Giaci crying, rebelling, and flailing his arms around while trying to run away from Shipu. Unperturbed, she would redirect him back to his chair, over and over again, and then continue her requests.

"Let's get to work, Giaci," she'd say calmly.

When Giaci went downstairs with her, it wasn't silently. His crying pierced my ears and dragged me down into his torment with him. I couldn't tell what was worse: the relentless commands or the hours of screeches. The girls weren't big fans of his screaming either; they would either cover their ears or cry with him, from upstairs. The thought of quitting surfaced many times. When John and I discussed it, he reminded me it was for our son's benefit. I just couldn't see it, nor could I take it anymore.

We didn't see any positive progress coming from the daily visits, and by the end of the first week, I couldn't even stay in the house during his sessions. I decided to put one twin in a baby-carrying sling over my chest and the other twin in the double stroller with Lauren. I had to get us out of the house. As the door clicked shut behind us and I pushed the double stroller onto the sidewalk, we could all still hear Giaci whine.

What kind of mother am I? I thought as I walked away, leaving my son with a stranger who was causing him distress. Lauren looked disgruntled; she knew something wasn't sitting well with me. At least the twins were satisfied just to be out in the fresh air, experiencing the world around them. Our walk was just as much to get them out of the house as it was for me to have some space to cry without them seeing my face. I cried for the entire walk around the block.

To avoid seeing the neighbours, I kept my head down and let the sobs silently seep from me. My life was so out of control, and I couldn't stop the madness. These sessions seemed to make the days worse, not better. My head knew that this had to be done, but my heart ached. With every step, I tried to rationalize what was happening in my home, telling myself that this was just like when a baby receives their first shots. It's for their own good, for their health and well-being. I was just doing what had to be done for my son's well-being.

I tried to justify it this way the entire walk around the block. And then, around the block again. I just kept imagining the unimaginable suffering happening in my house.

After twenty minutes of walking, I took the girls to our backyard to play on the swing set for another twenty minutes. Then I headed back inside the house with the girls.

"You okay, Mommy?" Lauren said, sensing my apprehension over going back into the house. "Can we walk tomorrow, too?" She turned her head to look at me, probably noticing my glossy eyes.

"Yes, of course we can, honey," I said.

It didn't matter that these walks were boring and drawn out; my little Lauren knew that we needed to get out of the house. She was always pulling me back to sanity.

As we entered the house, I braced myself, knowing that I would hear Giaci gasp for air between cries, but this time, I didn't hear anything. My heart dropped. Why didn't I hear crying? Then I heard Shipu say, "Good boy, Giaci."

I tiptoed farther into the house in disbelief. I didn't want to disrupt or stop any of the positivity I was hearing. Then I heard a mellifluous sound. My body involuntarily jolted, and I fell over as I was taking off my shoes. My heart stopped.

"Hi, Shipu," said a little angelic voice that sounded like heaven flowing from my basement. Was this Giaci's voice? It had to be—there was no one else there with him other than Shipu. The voice was soft and clear. He was responding with words, not tears or tantrums. I heard his sweet, delightful voice fully for the first time with Shipu.

I yearned to hear more.

"Way to go, Giaci! Nice job. High five!" Shipu said with a satisfied tone. The soft smack of their hands hitting each other ever so gently followed.

Numb, I continued listening, hoping to hear more from my little boy, but as usual, Shipu ended the session with "All done." At least this session had ended on a positive note.

I was still standing in the entryway and started helping the twins take off their shoes. That done, I asked Lauren to wait on the couch with her sisters while I ran downstairs to check on Giaci. Words escaped me as I fixated on Shipu, who had a big smile on her face. Her teeth were chalk white; I'd never seen her smile this big before.

"We had a good session today," she said.

These words echoed in my head. I froze in disbelief, unable to speak;

all the strength I had was focused on composing myself. I wanted to leap with joy and excitement, but I knew that such celebrations were premature. I didn't want to overreact over a single good session. Yet I was aware of the magnitude of this progress. The sun was starting to peer through the dark clouds, warming my cheeks with its glow. I smiled at Shipu, who could almost certainly see my tears.

"Thank you" were the only words my wobbly voice could muster.

She reciprocated by showing off her bright smile yet again as she put on her coat, pulling her long hair out from under it. She slipped on her shoes, grabbed her oversized black bag, and gave me a heartfelt goodbye that oozed confidence and reflected the day's achievement.

When Shipu left, Giaci didn't run back upstairs as he usually did. He stayed in the therapy area downstairs, sitting on the couch.

"Buddy, do you want to come up?" I asked.

He didn't answer. He sat on the green leather couch without moving or making a sound, so I didn't insist.

After leaving him alone for a few minutes, I went back down to check on him, still unable to read what he was thinking or feeling. Was he just so tired of crying and fighting all the demands that Shipu put on him? Or was he starting to understand that if he responded to a request, he would learn to communicate? I didn't know the answer because his cute little face seemed expressionless and depleted in that moment.

At the end of the session, he was lethargic. I sat down beside him silently and wrapped my shaking arms around him, holding him securely. Tears filled my eyes again. I wished I could take all of Giaci's struggles away. I wished that I had the power to make that happen.

If only I could snap my fingers and magically make all his struggles disappear.

But I didn't have magical powers.

Then I thought about God again—the only one who could make all the troubles in my life disappear. So why wouldn't He? I continued to cradle Giaci in my embrace, loving him with every bit of my existence, and wondered why God wouldn't answer my prayers and guide Giaci to a greater understanding of the world around him.

I was angry and exhausted. When I looked at Giaci lying in the crook of my arm, subdued from the day's mental tug-of-war, I gave him an extra squeeze. I wanted to give him some of my strength to help him gear up for the next day. With whatever armour we could find, whatever energy we could muster, we would keep learning together.

EIGHTEEN

"His Hearing Is Fine"

Hiring Shipu was a small step forward in admitting that Giaci was autistic, but that acknowledgement still didn't leave the house. The thought of admitting this stinging truth to the outside world chilled me. I wasn't ready.

The biggest roadblock was that autism was hard to explain to others. It is a complex developmental condition that presents differently in every individual. My son appeared normal physically, but cognitively he behaved very differently from other children.

His keen ability to spell large words had dissipated over the last year. He used to go to the fridge and spell big words with the magnetic letters, but he didn't do that anymore. It just stopped. He wasn't even interested in the letters. Instead, he was stuck in a repetitive action, whether it was flapping his hands and running or spinning with one of his toys in an odd, repetitive manner.

I had felt so excited that my son could do extraordinary things like spell big words by the age of two. But now he wasn't demonstrating any extraordinary abilities at all; rather, he was lacking basic social verbal skills.

My terror of the unknown resulted in my own struggle to connect with the world around me. I wasn't willing to accept that he wasn't going to be able to converse with me. I feared being viewed as a bad parent, and that others would pity us. *Poor Giaci, poor Rita.* If I didn't mention anything to anyone, then my son wouldn't be treated differently, or so I thought.

I wasn't sure when I became so engrossed in this cover-up, but I knew there had been a shift within me. I had gone from being a trusting, cheerful, naive, and confident person to being this shell of a woman that was filled with rage, fear, resentment, insecurity, and defeat. *I didn't plan for this* was all I heard repeating in my head.

I dreaded family events. Pretending all was well took a lot of energy.

Whenever we had family get-togethers, I tried to get out of them. Whether it was a birthday party or holiday dinner, I devised any excuse I could to not go. My brain often manipulated my body into getting sick. I had stomach pains and felt like vomiting.

"Do we have to go, John?" I whined one evening after he had gotten home from the construction site. We were getting ready to have Easter Sunday dinner at John's parents' house, but we were both exhausted from being up with Giaci the night before. I was pressed up against the bathroom door, watching John wash his hands after a long day.

"We have to," he said unconvincingly. "They're expecting us."

We were primed and conditioned to be respectful and to always show up for family affairs. Still, I groaned as I walked away from John, hoping that my sulking would change his mind.

I sifted through my closet to find an appropriate Easter outfit and settled on black dress pants and a spring-flowered blouse. I was already figuring out what the kids would wear. They were downstairs playing, so I called them up to get dressed. They'd have to be dressed up too, which wouldn't be a problem for Lauren or the twins. Giaci, though, had a hard time wearing tighter pants or any stiff shirt. If he had his way, he'd wear his comfy grey jogging pants and cotton T-shirt every day.

When John didn't give into my groan, I gave him my best drawn-out whine. "I reeeeally don't want to go," I shouted from the closet.

I knew that I couldn't disappoint family; they'd never let me live it down if I didn't show up for Easter, but part of me thought we could play up a stomach flu. A fever! Anything.

"Ri, I already told them we're coming. We don't have to stay long, but we have to go," he insisted, knowing the unspoken rules that applied to us.

The teachings of my upbringing—to always comply with expectations and be obedient—played on repeat in my mind. Cultural obligations overpowered me. It was as if I had lost a battle that was beyond my control. I didn't dare rebel. The thought of having to go to yet another dinner the next day with my side of the family also weighed on me.

Without any other options, I forced the actress in me to emerge. I had to put on a facade because I didn't dare show any hint of defeat or failure as a parent.

Before leaving, I gave my daughters a pep talk in the driveway.

"Girls, we need to always take care of Giaci together. Don't leave your brother for a minute, okay?" I pleaded as if our lives depended on it. In a way, they sort of did.

Lauren, always eager to please, didn't hesitate to say, "Yes, Mommy!"

Even the twins, who were three, understood my request and nodded.

My heart ached that the pressure of keeping our secret and the need to be a helicopter mom was also placed on my girls. I never meant to force them into this role, but I had nowhere to go and no one else to turn to. My only calming thought was that they wouldn't know any other reality; they were born into this one.

Once we got to Nonna and Nonno's house, I could tell that the girls were "on." Lauren's eyes zeroed in on the door, as if preparing for whatever waited inside, and the twins were quieter than usual. They were getting their heads in the game and ready to sacrifice playing with their cousins in order to be soldier nannies.

Giaci was oblivious to the tension around him; he was just focused on the fact that he would soon be devouring Nonna Carolina's homemade lasagna, his favourite food. There was no point having a pep talk with Giaci because he wouldn't be able to understand the conversation.

Family gatherings always had a hint of exhaustion tied to them, mainly because we ate too much and talked for hours. But they were still beautiful times we could spend together to celebrate life and family. As soon as the door to the kitchen swung open, the room smelled of rich Italian foods, pumped with acidic tomato sauce and savoury, stretchy mozzarella. I was sure John was already salivating at the smell of the lamb chops that had been marinating throughout the day and were now ready to sear on the grill. Memories of childhood family dinners washed over me and nearly knocked me over. The smell triggered my "on" button, and together, John, the girls, Giaci and I braced ourselves to walk into our new normal.

As soon as we entered the house, everyone greeted each other with a "*Buona Pasqua*"—Happy Easter—and we took off our shoes at the door. Nonna Carolina approached to receive hugs and kisses from the grandkids. I guided Giaci in her direction. She scooped him up and smacked a kiss on his cheek. He didn't seem fazed, and as soon as she plopped him back down on the tile floor, he ran off to the living room to watch TV. The girls all said their hellos and ran off right behind their brother, as directed.

As soon as Giaci was in front of the television, Lauren dove in front of him to find his favourite cartoon channel. The twins sat beside him, ready to help him if he needed anything. They knew that if Giaci was approached or spoken to, they would jump in to answer for him.

Seeing that Giaci was safe with his sisters, I made my rounds to greet family members I hadn't seen in months. It was nice interacting with them, but the cloud of worry and the fear of anyone learning that there was something wrong with my son still hovered over me.

I constantly peeked over to check on the kids. They were all still watching cartoons. Then one of the cousins asked Giaci, "What are you watching?"

I knew Giaci would have trouble processing this question, as he was too occupied by the action on the TV. "He didn't hear you," I said over the sound of *Duck Tales* playing.

"Are you sure he doesn't have a hearing problem? Have you had him checked?" my brother-in-law stepped in to ask. I was caught off guard.

"His hearing is fine," I snapped back.

He wasn't satisfied with my answer, though, and proceeded to clap his hands behind Giaci's head. It resonated in my ears from the other room. Giaci was in his happy place, watching a video he'd seen a million times before, anticipating the actions of the animated ducks. He didn't even flinch.

"See? He didn't hear that! He didn't even move." My brother-in-law said it like it was a valid assessment of my child's hearing.

I shrugged it off. "He's just really into his cartoons, so he isn't listening to anything else. His hearing is fine. I had it checked."

My own hearing was drowned out by the sound of my heart pounding in my head. Were we slowly being discovered? I could tell that he had more to say, but we were being called to the table to eat. I'm sure they knew something was off.

Twenty of us sat around the table filled with all the Easter specials—an antipasto of cheese and cured meats with fresh bread and olives. I made sure to keep Giaci beside me so I could monitor his manners. The girls sat near us too as plates of lasagna were served. The never-ending meal, with three kinds of meat and fish, overfilled the table. To Italians, breaking bread and eating bountiful meals together is an expression of love.

After two big plates of lasagna, Giaci was done. He was squirming out of his seat, wanting to go back to the living room and watch cartoons again. He'd had enough. I tried to hold him off so that he could eat the next course, but it was impossible. For fear of a tantrum erupting, I just released him.

Everyone was busy eating and chatting, so it seemed like no one really paid attention to Giaci's escape. Once the girls had finished their meals, they went to join their brother, and I prolonged my "everything is fine" performance with more small talk.

I counted down the seconds until I could wipe "Actress Rita" off of my face, but there were protocols when dealing with big family gatherings. I knew that after espresso, and the Italian desserts like cannoli and tiramisu, it would be the appropriate time to excuse ourselves.

I took my first full breath in the van ride home, and as soon as I walked through the door at home, I ran to the washroom to rinse the day away. I wiped off the hours of exhaustion and watched a stale version of myself flush down the drain. Actress Rita existed only when I needed her to, and I had to give her a break before she reappeared at my parents' house the next day for Easter Monday.

I looked at the Authentic Rita in the mirror. Her eyes were puffy from pretending; her hands sore from clutching at what used to be. She looked so different, paralyzed by a fear of judgment.

How much longer could I keep Actress Rita in my back pocket? She was fading away so quickly, and I worried that one day I'd reach for her, and she'd have disappeared completely.

NINETEEN

I Need Help!

As I waited to see my family doctor, a flyer pinned to the bulletin board in the waiting room caught my eye: "Feeling sad? Need someone to talk to? Call Tanner at the Wellness Centre."

The flyer made it seem so simple, as if Tanner could make all my problems—my struggles with acceptance—just go *poof!* and disappear. The thought of having a professional make sense of the jumbled mess inside my head and maybe pull me out of it was tempting. I dug through my purse to find a scrap of paper and quickly wrote down the number.

I gripped that little piece of paper on my way into Dr. Chang's office. I thought it might be a good idea to ask her about Tanner at the Wellness Centre and the help I knew I needed.

"I just…haven't been feeling like myself," I explained to her. I kept it simple, not releasing too much information, but still indicating that my mental state wasn't what it once had been. "I saw the flyer in your waiting room, with Tanner, the counsellor. Can I make an appointment with him?"

"Well, it does sound like seeking help might be a good idea. If after getting counselling you still aren't feeling like yourself, come back to see me. We could revisit possibly prescribing meds," she said, like it was nothing.

I didn't know how I felt about taking medication for my sadness. I didn't think I was *there* yet. "Thanks, Dr. Chang," I said. "I'll keep you posted."

My ego would barely allow me to seek help; my personal ship had run aground. It was embarrassing, and I felt like a failure. The sadness was dark, powerful, and depressing.

After leaving the doctor's office, I sat in the car and clutched my cellphone, having already punched in the number. *Just do it. Just dial*, I kept repeating, hoping that if I flinched an inch, the number would just magically go through without any real effort on my part. *Do you want your life to change?* Yes, of course I did. I wanted to be me again, happy and carefree. I wanted John and I to be us again, not drifting apart. I wanted to enjoy all my children.

I pressed *send* and let the phone ring.

Someone picked up. "Hello, Wellness Centre."

"Hi there. I'd like to make an appointment with Tanner."

* * *

On the day of the appointment with the counsellor, I was nervous. I tried to rationalize my fears. My son was working hard every day with Shipu, trying to find his voice, trying to interact with others, so the least I could do was sit in this dull grey room for him. It was my turn to get help, and John said it was a good idea too.

I looked around the room; framed credentials filled one wall, and a painting of a fall scene was displayed on the other. I thought about what I'd say to this stranger: "Hi, my son is autistic, and that makes me feel really helpless"? That was probably *exactly* what I would say if I could even manage to get the words out. I knew that I couldn't bear the sadness that consumed me anymore. I struggled to accept our life as it was. Something within me had to change. I was looking for guidance on how to move beyond sadness and feelings of failure and to learn how to fumble toward acceptance.

I sat there fidgeting and thinking for what felt like weeks before Tanner finally came in to greet me. I expected him to look like an old scientist, but instead he was middle-aged and dressed in comfortable clothes, like an average person. He even looked like a friend of John's, named Pat.

"Rita?" he asked in a mellow tone.

I straightened up.

"Nice to meet you. I'm glad you are here. Why don't we get started?" He extended his arm, as if to give the room a big embrace, and motioned for me to sit on the couch instead of the uncomfortable waiting-room-type chair. I took in his kindness and tried to let my ego go as I walked over to the black leather couch.

You're doing this for Giaci. For yourself. For your family.

"So, Rita, why did you come to see me?" Tanner asked.

I sat on the other end of that question, mulling over the answer I'd been chewing on for the last few days. I wanted it to come out elegantly and well thought out, but instead, I just burst out, "I need help! I don't know how to handle my son's autism diagnosis. I've lost myself and don't feel like I can be present for my family." I rambled and then cried as I opened the raw, bleeding wound that was carved into my spirit. "Can you help me?"

"Wow. Thank you for your honesty, Rita. I'm going to do my best to help you," he said. "How about we take a big breath? You're brave for coming to see me. Just now, you're telling me everything that you came in for; that was another brave thing." I felt like a child being coddled, but I'd never been more grateful for an emotional pat on the back from a stranger. I followed his lead and took a deep breath. It felt like the fullest breath I'd taken in nearly four years.

"Good. Now, do you want to tell me about the diagnosis? When did you find out?"

With that, I proceeded to tell Tanner about the official day of receiving the diagnosis.

* * *

It was on the day I met with child psychologist Dr. Gary. Just she and I met on this day. She was well respected and well known in our local autism community. We had been on her waitlist for two years, so when our time came up, I took Giaci to see her for our first visit. After her observations with my son, and me filling out all the questionnaires she provided, I met her in her office to go over the results.

That meeting wasn't at all like a parent–teacher interview, which is what I was accustomed to having when discussing a child's progress. This was very different. I sat tapping the arms of the chair in front of her metal desk as she explained her findings. This was the second psychological assessment my son had been given in his short life; the first was when he was three, which never mentioned autism. The assessment said Pervasive Developmental Disorder, which I didn't know at the time meant that he was on the autism spectrum. And now, with Giaci at age five, we were doing another assessment.

Even though I knew that my son had autism now, it was hard to listen as she explained where he was situated on the autism spectrum. I gazed at her with tight, grim lips. My jaw clenched as I grew heated, and my shoulders took on a hardened, defensive posture. I wasn't angry with her, as she was just the messenger; I was angry with how our lives had changed.

"Will Mr. Miceli be joining us today?" she asked from behind the pages of her notebook, her upturned brown eyes resting behind round wire-rimmed glasses.

"No. He's unable to make it, so we can proceed," I answered with an impatient tone. I hadn't even told John about this meeting. I wanted to spare him from having to hear our son's assessment results yet again. It was hard enough to hear the assessment results the first time, and John had so much work to do. I was ready to take the knockout punch for both of us.

"All right, then! We can begin," Dr. Gary said in a blasé manner. These meetings must have been so routine for her. It was not what *I* was used to doing; however, I did cringe at the idea of her having to sit through this day after day.

She spoke in a clear, regular pattern, like a medical doctor would before giving you bad news. She started with the background information, which was basically all the information I had provided about my son, and then proceeded to tell me the names of the tests she had administered, including the Childhood Autism Rating Scale (CARS). Then came the results. I adjusted myself in the uncomfortably stiff, ill-fitting chair, trying to find a position to hold.

"Giaci's overall adaptive behaviour at home was within the mild deficit range of almost two-and-a-half years behind expectations," she read like she was reading off an order at a fast-food restaurant. All I heard was that he was functioning at half his age. She also implied that this gap would most likely increase as my child grew. Dr. Gary continued glancing between her papers and me, perhaps expecting to see a reaction on my face, but there was none. I was stiff, hard, and cold.

Her words began to sound like those of Charlie Brown's teacher, Miss Othmar.

Wah, wah, wah-wah.

"Your son's results were consistent with moderate Autistic Disorder."

I snapped back to reality. "Okay, so he's in the middle? Not severe, but not mild either? So, is that good? Bad? Does it really matter?" I willed myself to an inner haven, away from the difficult words I had to hear. Yet nothing could protect me from the final blow.

"Well, his IQ score is below 70, which means he is functioning in the mentally retarded range."

My quivering bottom lip pressed against my upper lip in an effort to stabilize both. I was barely hanging on to the contents of my stomach.

Noticing a change, a sudden thawing of my expressionless face, she added, "This is a scientific term that is used in assessments only, so please don't be upset by it. It's the same as saying he has an intellectual disability. It is used only in psychological assessments."

I wandered out of my head to seek refuge elsewhere again. I couldn't listen to her anymore. The seat under me felt uncomfortable, the heat in my face flushed, my heart raced with agitation. Dr. Gary was gentle, though, and tried to reassure me.

"An assessment is just a snapshot of your son. It doesn't tell us everything about him. It's a standardized test."

I felt overwhelmed. I was losing control. I had to move this meeting along. I couldn't sustain the blows of the words used to describe my little boy.

"Thank you, Dr. Gary. I know it's your job to complete these tests. I'm so grateful for your time, but I have to go." I stood. "I'm late to pick up my children." I clenched my heavy purse with weak arms, bowed my head, and proceeded to the door.

"I understand. I'll be sending you a few copies in the mail," she explained as she escorted me to the hallway.

I hurried out the door and bolted to the van. I heard her voice echo in my head as I crumbled onto the seat in the minivan. I don't remember the drive home.

* * *

"And now, here I am, Tanner, with pieces of me shattered on the inside. I don't know who I am anymore. I just cry all the time, and I can't even remember what a smile feels like," I said. He nodded as if he had heard this all before.

"I understand. It's understandable to be sad. What you're feeling is grief. You are mourning the son you thought you had, Rita. You need to mourn for however long you need to mourn, and that is different for everyone."

As he spoke, my eyes filled up with tears. It was like he was giving me permission to be sad about my son's disability.

It made sense to me now.

In that moment, I realized that I had been mourning quietly by myself without receiving any condolences or support from anyone, because no one knew.

"Rita, you cannot let a standardized test define your son. He is who he is and who he was meant to be. He is still your son, and your love for him will never falter."

My tears turned into a sobbing lament.

He was right, and I had to release the desire of wanting it to be different. I could not be stuck in this mental space anymore. This is how my son was meant to be. I could not control or change him. I needed to understand and accept him as he was. He was beautiful in every way, and I needed to see that.

It made sense to me now.

TWENTY

Ambiguous Loss

My sessions with Tanner continued to force me to dig deep, and once I realized that I was grieving, it truly helped me move forward.

It wasn't that my son had died a physical death. If that had been the case, there would have been a funeral. People would have brought flowers, cards and fruit baskets to my door and left condolences. That type of mourning has its protocols, but this type does not. What John and I were experiencing was not a physical loss, because our son was alive and strong. He was vibrant and present.

No, our loss was more ambiguous. It stared at me through Giaci's eyes when he couldn't find his words, yet it disappeared any time he achieved something new. Every time the loss was within reach so we could deal with it, it dissolved between my fingers. It wasn't tangible. No one else could understand it; *we* barely could.

Tanner's main job was to guide me through these feelings of grief and mourning. I devoured every piece of literature he gave me on the topic of ambiguous loss, hoping to ease the pain of a disoriented mind. In doing so, I learned that it occurs without closure or understanding. This type of loss leaves a person searching for answers, thus complicating and delaying the process of grieving. It often results in unresolved grief. In this context, it made sense that I felt like I was living on a roller coaster—one minute on a high filled with hope and thoughts of a bright future, and the next plummeting to the ground. My days strapped me in tight, but I could never fully brace myself for the motion sickness that each minute brought.

Tanner also helped me understand how John and I mourned differently. John was much better at accepting that our son was who he was meant to be, whereas I wanted to change Giaci. My daily task was to fight all the things I felt needed changing for our son.

John focused his attention on working to provide the funds to pay for the therapies our son needed to improve his life—whatever that life would be. John shed tears after reading the results from Dr. Gary's report when I gave it to him.

Coping differently didn't make one way better than the other. We were both in survival mode and had our roles to fulfill. So, taking out our frustration or anger on each other would only weaken us, and I wasn't going to let that happen. We needed every ounce of strength to lift each other up.

Next, I read about Pauline Boss, the researcher who first coined the term *ambiguous loss* in the late 1970s. She was studying the families of soldiers who went missing in action, and she found that they struggled with grieving when there was no body to bury. Ambiguity is confusing, and when it's difficult to make sense of the situation, feelings of helplessness, depression and anxiety are the result. That described me precisely.

Holding two opposing ideas in one's mind at the same time, Boss explained, is physically and emotionally exhausting, particularly when that state persists for a long time. This was what I was living.

Boss also explained that among the families she studied, their grief remained frozen in place unless the families were able to reconstruct their own identities and roles.

I started to think about my own life in the context of Pauline Boss's advice: "To address ambiguous loss with patience, care, and compassion," I needed to be patient, caring, and compassionate with myself. I just didn't know how to get there. Instead, I festered in anger.

I brought this up to Tanner at one of our sessions.

"I'm angry, Tanner. I'm furious that this happened to me, my son and our family. Why did this happen, and why are there no answers?"

He responded calmly, "It seems like maybe your anger is complicated, with a lot of blame you're putting on yourself."

I nodded, dismayed. Maybe I did blame myself.

"Is it my fault? What did I do? I carried him in my belly and have nurtured him from the first breath he took. I have always been loving, yet he remains distant."

Tanner never gave me any certainties; he only offered more questions. "Do you *feel* like it was something you did?"

"Maybe. I carried him, so maybe I gave him autism." These words were barely above a whisper. Guilt gripped my throat.

"Rita, did you give him green eyes? Did you have control over that?"

"No, that was not something I controlled," I responded.

"Did you give him brown hair?" he asked.

"No." I sank in my seat. "I couldn't take it if I were the reason he's as isolated as he is."

"Does he look isolated?" Tanner asked, which flustered me.

"Of course he looks isolated! He can't communicate with anyone. That must be so lonely!" I burst out.

Tanner nodded along, jotting down notes in his book. "It must be lonely for you too. Do you have other ways of communicating?"

This question took me by surprise. Did I have other ways of communicating with Giaci? Or was I so caught up in getting him to communicate in my language I couldn't see any alternatives? "Are there other ways of communicating?" he asked.

"Yes, I believe there are other ways of communicating," I said. "When he smiles at me, I know he is happy. When he hugs me, I know he loves me and feels loved." I sat up. "When he laughs after being tickled, I know he is having fun."

I was understanding the direction of his questions.

"Exactly." Tanner's voice was like a gentle hand on my shoulder—

comforting, yet a firm nudge to move forward. "Good work today. Let's revisit the celebrations and beauty in all the shared moments next week," he said, and wrote down more homework for me to dive into.

I took the prescription to heart, starting with analyzing and deconstructing the crushing guilt I felt.

* * *

When I got home, I dove into the homework I was given about the historical information on the "refrigerator mother." In the 1950s and '60s, Bruno Bettelheim, one of the first child development specialists to focus on autism, advanced this explanation for its origins. Bettelheim had spent time in a Nazi concentration camp and believed he saw parallels between the behaviour of camp prisoners and that of autistic children. This led him to reason that autism was a psychological disturbance arising from detached and "frigid" mothering—like how prisoners reacted to the intense authority of camp guards. *Unfair!*

It took decades for the medical community to listen to the few voices such as Dr. Bernard Rimland, Dr. Erick Schopler, and the mothers themselves who had been challenging this unfounded theory of "mother-blame" since the early '60s. Maybe Bettelheim's theory was more about him having been a prisoner than it was about mothers.

Although discredited by medical consensus, the refrigerator mother theory revived my fear that this was all my fault. I had hugged and kissed my babies constantly, offering never-ending love. They were smothered with affection. Did that sound like a "lack of maternal warmth"? How could I be compared to frigid concentration camp guards? Was my son a prisoner—*my* prisoner? My mind raced at the devastating thought that I would have to shoulder the blame.

I had carried Giaci for nine months. He grew inside me! I ate responsibly, took my vitamins, and made sure to follow every pregnancy health tip I could find. Where had I gone wrong?

All this reading didn't soothe my worries at all; if anything, it made my nightly outbursts worse. Now I couldn't hide my loud sobbing from John.

"Rita?" John said groggily as he rolled over one night. "Are you crying?"

I whimpered, and he held me while I searched for the right words. "Why did this happen to our son?" I asked, but I knew John had no answers.

He rubbed my back and kept repeating, "Shh. I don't know."

"What could I have done? I must have done something wrong. I feel like it's my fault."

"Rita, it wasn't you. You did nothing wrong. You have done everything right, and you continue to do everything right. This is just how Giaci was meant to be, and you have to accept that." There it was again: his complete acceptance that this was "just the way things were."

"I can't. I just can't," I mumbled, but John's breathing had already shifted back from chest to belly breath. He was asleep again.

"I just can't," I said to myself as I rolled back over.

*　*　*

The next morning, I woke with a familiar recurring fear: that I'd have to take care of my child for the rest of my life. This wasn't a new worry. Over the years, John and I had discussed the possibility many times. John had accepted this early on and planned for our son's future, knowing that we would always have to care for him.

"We'll make sure we have the funds he'll need to have constant care, and I know our girls will never abandon him." He attempted to soothe me yet again, but it was never enough. In fact, it was even worse because I worried that the girls would resent us for leaving them with this responsibility.

Now, when I lifted myself out of bed and padded to the bathroom, I looked at a sun-faded portrait of myself in the mirror. My skin was dull, lacking colour in my cheeks. I had thought the sessions with Tanner would help, but they were just bringing all my fears to the surface. I wasn't ready to confront them all at the same time. But maybe I needed to. It was heavy and it was time.

Giaci's abilities were limited: he couldn't express his wants and needs. He couldn't tell me about his day. At this rate, he could never live independently. That part hit me the hardest.

It was another loss, the loss of never moving him into a college or university dorm one day, the loss of never watching him move in with a family of his own.

As I thought of Giaci's life of solitude, I sobbed into the sink. At least for now I was right there with him, feeling trapped and alone in unimaginable torment. But what would happen to him in the future, if or when I was no longer around?

In *Ambiguous Loss*, Pauline Boss writes, "An ambiguous loss can freeze people in place so they can't move on with their lives. Ambiguous loss is the most stressful loss people can face."

Reading this brought on an even greater sense of dread. Autism is lifelong. There was no closure for me in this fact, only an unknown future. The only solution was resilience.

I had always considered myself resilient, but was I?

I ran through a checklist of my latest qualities: an inability to bounce back; a tendency to isolate myself from others; and a refusal to ask anyone for help or to admit there is a problem.

These qualities did not add up to a resilient person. John was a resilient person. He trudged on with his days and accepted each of our kids for who they were. He never wavered or broke down. John was our rock, while I felt like the crumbling clay beneath him.

On the other hand, John didn't have to endure the long days the same way I did. This thought felt like a breakthrough, so I ran to the kitchen drawer, pulled out a notepad and wrote it down. I'd started this habit after my visits with Tanner; it seemed to help keep my thoughts straight before our next meeting. While frantically scribbling, I imagined being someone else—a person who could see me from the outside. I wrote:

Rita—you're not yourself these days. You're tired. Exhausted by the struggles of living with four little ones so close in age. You feel like a single mom because John works so much, and it puts even more stress on you.

But there's more. There's something you're hiding.

I know it's not easy to ask for help, but we're all human beings, and we all need to ask for help. If you're not comfortable with letting me in, that's okay. I'll wait, and when you're ready to talk, I'll be here ready to listen. No judgment. Know that I'm here for you whenever you need me.

You're strong.

You're resilient.

When I put down the pen, it felt as if a long-lost friend had just dropped by for a visit. She still lived deep inside me, and just that brief visit made me feel like I was an inch closer to getting her back for good.

TWENTY-ONE

The "Cut-Off" Age

Visits with Tanner were not as often now. I really did feel like he'd helped me sort out the many questions that filled my head. His homework exercises were helpful too.

One quote from my reading that helped me understand my grief over losing the "perfect" little boy I thought I had was from Elisabeth Kübler-Ross and David Kessler's *On Grief and Grieving*:

> The reality is that you will grieve forever. You will not "get over" the loss of a loved one; you will learn to live with it. You will heal and you will rebuild yourself around the loss you have suffered. You will be whole again, but you will never be the same. Nor should you be the same, nor would you want to.

I was learning to live with it, and I was now "better enough" to take matters into my own hands again. Giaci was five and a half years old and still working with Shipu. Their sessions were play-based. He was mastering skills like repetition, pointing, one-word and two-word vocalizations, and it wasn't a battle like the first week was. Giaci enjoyed their sessions together and was thriving because it was fun. Now he was able to answer simple questions about things like his name, his family members' names, his address, and other personal information, and I had many more things on my list that needed to be taught.

John and I paid Shipu privately. It was costly and stretched our family finances thin. We were still waiting for the government program, which would have alleviated our financial burdens. But this program ended at age six regardless of when Giaci would get picked up.

Now we were faced with a different kind of fight: the fight over government funding.

It had been almost a year since Giaci was added to the waitlist for services and programming that the government offered to children with autism. We were running out of time, as the "cut-off" age for these services was six years old.

When a letter arrived from the government service provider, indicating that in a week there would be a meeting about Intensive Behavioural intervention services for my son at a centre nearby, I was prepared to go and make sure these services started right away. I believed that once the program began, I would get additional help for Giaci, and more behavioural intervention to help him catch up.

* * *

When I arrived at the meeting in the local not-for-profit children's centre, I signed in at the table near the door. A woman stood behind it, and I was finally able to put a face to at least one of the voices I'd spoken to on the phone almost every day. I peered up at her after signing in and decided to give her my pageant-winning smile. She wouldn't recognize this cheery mama now.

"Is this meeting about starting services?" I asked. "Will families be given a start date tonight?" I grinned, hoping to get the answer I wanted.

"Tonight is an information night," she said in monotone, just like she did over the phone. "There will be a discussion about what will happen before it starts." She waved as if to shoo me into the room.

Remembering this sort of defeat from my many phone calls, I followed her direction to the table.

At the table, two other mothers and one father sat in swivel chairs facing the screen that displayed the agenda:

1. Introductions
2. What Is ABA (Applied Behaviour Analysis)?
3. IBI (Intensive Behaviour Intervention)
4. Behaviour Teams
5. Parent Coaching

I twisted my ring and looked around the room, noticing the other parents shifting in their seats too. The meeting started right on time, and as soon as the lights dimmed, the speakers—Jeff and Rino—introduced themselves. They were behaviour clinicians on the early intervention autism team and had the four of us parents introduce ourselves. I started to clue into where this meeting was going when one of the speakers said, "We'll be having a number of meetings together before the in-home therapy begins for your child."

In-home therapy for my child.

Woohoo. It's about time.

The first parent to speak was Sarah.

She started the conversation with a strong, confrontational statement: "My son is almost six years old, which means he'll be getting cut from these services soon." Everyone looked around at each other, unsure of what to say as her steaming blue eyes nearly burned a hole through the projector screen.

Marni spoke up: "My son is in the same situation," she said. Her deep red curls echoed her anger, and it was all directed at Jeff and Rino.

The rest of us realized that we too were in the same situation. These parents were ready to pounce, and I could see a hint of concern beneath Jeff and Rino's stoic expressions. Without responding to the first two women, Jeff pointed at me to indicate that I could go next.

"Hello, my name is Rita, and my son is five years old. I'm hoping that we're here tonight to get behaviour therapy started for my son," I said.

Jeff continued to nod as the lone father introduced himself, expressing the same anxiety over getting services started right away.

The meeting continued with Jeff and Rino sidestepping our concerns and elaborating on the parent coaching that was to come. They talked for two long hours.

When they were done, it was clear that everyone in the room felt depleted; our eyelids were heavy and our bodies sank in the chairs. We were all frustrated with the delays in service, and now even more expectations were being put upon us, such as having to come to meetings like this and doing hours and hours of mandatory parent coaching. We shook our heads in unison, all annoyed we'd have to take on even more work than we were already doing. They indicated that we, the parents, had to actively participate in team meetings, had to take the training on ABA/IBI, which was hours of learning, *and* we had to work with and alongside our child and provide data collection—all this in addition to everything we were doing as parents and breadwinners.

Intensive behaviour intervention (IBI) consists of a variety of procedures drawn from the field of ABA. The main goal of ABA is to give children with autism the skills necessary to learn naturally from their homes, schools, and community environments. These goals are achieved through environmental manipulations, modelling, shaping, reinforcement, feedback, and other behavioural strategies. The main difference between IBI and ABA is the level of intensity, with IBI more focused and directed.

In the upcoming parent-coaching sessions, we'd all learn strategies to help our sons—all the attendees tonight had sons with autism—but we were all spent, with lives that were overwhelming before we'd even walked through the door. Each of us had already put in a full day of work before attending this meeting, so the fact that they were loading us up with more work was maddening.

On the way out, two other moms and I sparked a conversation in the hallway.

"How long have you been on the waitlist for services?" Sarah asked.

"Too long," I responded.

Marni jumped in. "I'm most worried about the cut-off age. My son won't get much help if we're cut off," she said.

Then Sarah informed us of the one potential bright light.

"Have you guys added your name to the class-action lawsuit that's fighting this age restriction?" she asked.

A class-action lawsuit is a type of lawsuit where one of the parties is a group of people—which we were as parents of children with autism—who are represented collectively.

Marni and I exchanged glances and shook our heads.

"Who do I call?" I nearly screamed. Finally, a way I could take control!

We exchanged phone numbers, and Sarah said she would text us the information. This was the beginning of a friendship driven by our convictions and desire to act for the greater good. This age discrimination against our children had started a fire in us.

While at work the next day, I had a hard time teaching my students. My focus was on the class-action lawsuit. As soon as I got home, I called the lawyer to get more details and to add us to the group. Even though it didn't take much effort to make the call, it felt like I was jumping over a line, and that fuelled me. I heard an unfamiliar chant in my head, awakening an inner strength I didn't know I still had. *Yes!*

The parent-coaching sessions began the next week, and after each one, there was still no indication of when the behaviour team would start working with Giaci. I was grateful that John and I had the means to provide Giaci with a therapist like Shipu who could keep him on track, but not everyone was so lucky.

Even though the meetings were for us parents, they weren't particularly helpful because we wanted to see direct services to our sons. But we had to attend. Getting my son into the government Intensive Behaviour Intervention program was critical for helping him gain additional skills and address behaviours, so I had to follow their process.

My busy school and child-minding schedule made going to the

meetings especially draining, but every time I got there, I was uplifted by the connections I made. Collaborating with the other parents gave me the support I had been lacking.

Not only did these meetings give me information I needed, but they also gave me friends who understood what I was going through. With Sarah and Marni, I didn't have to pretend that I wasn't struggling. I didn't have to put on a performance or explain this new version of myself. For the first time in a long time, I felt like I belonged. Like I had purpose.

We all wanted to access this intervention for our sons immediately and for longer than the age six restriction. I felt like I'd started the advocating alone. But I wasn't alone anymore. I had backup.

TWENTY-TWO

Fired Up in the Courthouse

When Shipu announced she was getting married and moving away, we were happy for her but devastated for our family. We couldn't handle the thought of losing the therapist who'd helped Giaci progress so much. As always, my mind ran to the worst-case scenario: What would happen to Giaci without this intervention?

But then, in that crucial moment, we got word that the government program was starting up for our son, just as Shipu was leaving.

It was invigorating to have more than one person running his programming. With the government program, it was an entire team complete with instructor therapists, a senior therapist, and a clinical psychologist who would oversee Giaci's skill acquisition and development. But with Giaci already being five, we were left with only a year to reap the benefits of the program.

Of course, I didn't want it to end; that's why I joined forces with other parents like me to stop the Ontario government from discriminating based on age. As far as I was concerned, they couldn't cut our kids off from this funding.

* * *

"I booked us on the late bus to Toronto," Sarah said. "We can sleep on the bus and be there first thing in the morning." She had called early in the morning to disclose the details of our trip to Toronto for the class-action lawsuit that she, Marni, and I had signed on to.

She didn't waste time when it came to getting what she needed for her son. We were the same in that respect and it was refreshing to have an ally who was just as passionate as I was.

"You're the best. Thanks for doing that, Sarah." I took a breath. It was nice to have someone else check an item off my to-do list. "Did you read all of the paperwork from our lawyer?" I tried to keep my tone neutral, but disgust coiled around the words. "I still can't believe they want to cut our kids off so soon."

I could hear Sarah's breath creating a film of steam on her receiver. She wasn't one for mincing words or tucking emotions away. "It's outrageous!" she exclaimed. "Our sons need this therapy to learn the skills to be more independent. We want them to gain these skills now so they won't be a burden to society and to taxpayers later in life. How can they not see that?"

* * *

At the courthouse, nothing appeared to be accomplished. Legal counsel after legal counsel gabbed away but no decision was made about removing the age restriction. I wanted an immediate decision to continue services for life, but that didn't happen. Nothing was determined, which infuriated us with the lack of progress. The government didn't want to listen. According to them, research emphasized the need to treat children while they were young, so the age restriction was "justified." Not to us. Learning doesn't end at age six. We are constantly learning throughout life, so why would persons with autism be any different?

At one point, we were sitting on a wooden bench in the hallway prior to entering the courtroom. Sarah, with her elevated frustration, quickly jumped up from the bench, unable to settle, and started pacing outside the courtroom door. Marni and I remained sitting, staring at Sarah's movements as she stomped back and forth on the tile floor. Out of the corner of my eye, I noticed a man approaching us. He was neatly dressed in a navy pinstripe suit and pale pink tie. His dark hair was slicked back with gel, holding his government persona together.

When Sarah noticed him, she redirected her pouncing energy. "Are you representing the government in this case?" She trailed after him.

When he didn't answer, she carried out a one-sided conversation with pride. "I don't know how you can defend their side! How do you sleep?" Many people wouldn't understand how she could flail her arms and rant at a government lawyer or become so inflamed with rage that even her hair spiralled, but Marni and I could. Most mothers could.

"Look at her go," Marni whispered to me. "If anyone's going to get the job done, it's her." We watched our teammate in amazement and braced ourselves to be pulled in, but we wouldn't jump in unless she needed backup. This was her kill.

When the walking suit finally stopped to brave Sarah, she squinted and zeroed in like a mama lion who'd just been crossed. "This therapy is the only thing that can help our children." Sarah looked back at us to indicate our united front. "Why would you fight against the only services offered to our sons?"

The lawyer didn't respond. We couldn't tell if he was considering her words or simply dozing off.

Sarah, apparently exhausted by his lack of response, burned hotter.

"I hope to God that you don't ever have a child with autism because then you'll know first-hand the irreversible damage you're causing," she hissed.

When Sarah's rant finally ended, the dapper lawyer nodded as if to say *Are we done here?* With the lift of his brown leather briefcase, he continued into the courtroom with the entourage of other lawyers who had suddenly appeared behind him.

Watching them stride into the room, Sarah stood straight and proud until the door shut behind them. Then she caved in on herself. It wasn't easy holding that protective stance on her own. Marni and I both knew that feeling of defeat, so we ran to her side to help lift some of the weight off her. As she leaned into us, her glossy eyes emitted one tear at a time. Marni and I looked at each other as if we wanted to join her in her release.

No decision was made, so sporadic court visits to Toronto like this one continued for three years. They were emotionally draining, though it wasn't quite like the exhaustion we felt at home. This was different—this was getting close to the finish line, only to be knocked to the side by our opponent. The government lawyers were fighting dirty by indicating that ABA/IBI was not a medical treatment, so their case was that the government was not obligated to provide this at all for children with autism. We were supposed to be thankful that it was being offered up until age six. The opposing side, who was fighting for us, reiterated the enormous amount of research indicating that this was evidence-based, and it was beneficial at any age. The two sides would debunk the other's evidence, and it continued as a thumb war of back and forth. We all felt as if we were reduced to nothing when it came to dealing with the judicial system. We were just a case number, a conquest on the battlefield where they knew they had the upper hand.

* * *

I held out hope until I received a letter from our lawyer, who was representing many Ontario families in this class-action lawsuit. We had lost the case.

I was devastated. We had fought for three whole years. We had sat through all the legal jargon, with one side pleading their case and then the other side doing the same. We'd had to listen to testimony and arguments for hours and endure the annoying lack of progress, first for months, and then for years. We'd heard of countless children with autism being cut off from services. All were dropped right at age six—just like *our* sons had been.

After reading the letter, I let out a howl so loud I thought I'd wake the kids. I couldn't hold in my feeling of defeat, so I dialed John's cell number to tell him about the news in between sobs. This seemed to have finally kicked me down once and for all. There was no getting up from this.

But on the other end of the line, John sounded energized. He said the same thing he'd said so many times before: "Rita, we have been providing Giaci with this therapy privately. We are going to continue doing it. I'll continue to work seven days a week. We have to do what we have to do, and we'll get through this, too. I know the cost for this intervention is high for us, but we will do it."

For so long I had felt like we were ships passing each other in the night, off to different locations, sailing through opposing storms. The truth was that we'd been weathering the same storm this entire time; John was at the helm, trying to steer us to safety, while I was busy checking all the sails and tying the ropes. They were different tasks leading us to the same shining lighthouse.

"Thank you, honey. I needed that. I love you, John," I said. I spoke with my heart fully for what seemed like the first time in years. We'd loved each other through the good and the bad, just like our parents had taught us to. I wouldn't have wanted to run this ship with anyone but him and the rest of our crew.

I knew that not everyone was as lucky as we were. ABA/IBI therapy cost us about $50,000 a year in those days. It often cost people their marriages, their health, and their other children's extracurricular activities. I often wondered if our girls were getting enough attention, if their needs were being met, and if John and I could continue to endure the exhaustion and stress. John was working endless hours to meet our financial needs, and my heart hurt for those families that wouldn't be able to provide their children with the same much-needed therapists.

"I know we won't stop doing what we have to for our son," I continued, "but I hate the thought of leaving the others behind." I thought of Marni, of Sarah, of every other helpless parent out there who was desperately paddling alone in their boat, of those who had holes in the bottoms of their last life raft.

There were wrongs to be righted.

The fight in me hadn't died out just yet.

TWENTY-THREE

Getting a Haircut

As one battle fizzled, another ignited.

Some things were becoming easier for Giaci. Thanks to the intervention, he was getting things like expressing his wants, such as "I want waffles," or "I want tickles." He was interacting more and more with me, John, and his sisters. He was able to dress and undress himself. He could identify body parts and follow instructions. Each skill was broken down into small steps with slow introductions, like getting a haircut.

I remember how difficult it had been for Giaci to get a haircut in the beginning. For most young children, getting a haircut can be an uncomfortable experience filled with unease; for Giaci, it was complete sensory overload.

Italian superstition held that I couldn't cut my babies' hair until they were one year old; not following this custom could invite "bad luck." Whether I believed this or not, I followed this tradition honourably like a good Italian daughter and waited until shortly after Giaci's first birthday to have Nonno Vito cut Giaci's hair.

I brought baby Giaci into Dad's barbershop before I even knew I was dealing with autism, and by the time we sat him in the chair he was already fussing. Even though he would not sit still, and cried through the entire haircut, we both chalked it up to normal discomfort.

Thinking back on it now, I realize the magnitude of my son's sensory distress. There were the flickering lights, the uncomfortable nylon cape squeezing his little neck and blocking his view of his on-the-move hands, the strong smells of hair products and shaving cream, the cold water sprayed on his round head, and the snipping sounds of the scissors. He had to contend with the loud electric clipper brushing up the back of his neck and around his little ears, and countless other things that I wasn't aware of. They all piled up, resulting in too much sensory information to take in.

Those haircuts in Giaci's early years put my son in his own personal torture chamber. Dad was so patient and tried his best, but the back of Giaci's head wasn't always as straight as he would have liked.

Instinctively I began introducing Giaci to the *steps* of a haircut at the onset of getting a haircut. I thought this would be easiest done in the bathtub, because he was often distracted by the water and loved playing with his rubber ducky toys. At first, I would just show him the comb and allow him to touch its bristles and understand that it could not harm him.

Then, for the next few baths, I would comb his hair in the tub, stopping if he grew agitated. Being able to recognize Giaci's limits was an important step in getting him comfortable with the entire process. I'm not sure how I knew what to do, but my rule was to always use Giaci's boundaries as a guide. Even when I didn't know what to do, I trusted that he would show me what he did and didn't want.

And then I would creep up a little more each time.

After about a week of just combing, I introduced the scissors into his view. The scissors were a scarier object to Giaci than the comb, especially with their sharp edges. Words were unnecessary in the early years, as they would just complicate the situation. So, I started by cutting a piece of his hair myself, showing him his hair and clapping when he accepted this behaviour.

"Good job, buddy! You were so good!" I said, splashing the water around with him, showing him that this experience could be a fun one.

After months of building him up like this, I decided that he was ready for the full haircutting experience with Nonno Vito again—only this time, I had a few tricks up my sleeve.

We couldn't just jump right into cutting; we started with a visit. I brought Giaci to Dad's barber shop to just sit in the barber's chair. There were days and days of these visits. The cozy chair swivelled, which made Giaci giggle and bounce at the fun he could have in this space. This felt like a reward of its own.

Next, we had him sit on the chair and draped the cape over him for the added sensory experience. Giaci coped well with it now. There were a few visits in which John would model the behaviour we wanted—calmly getting his own haircut while Giaci watched. Step by step Giaci's tolerance increased, as did his understanding of the experience.

At almost six, he was "number one" (as Dad would say) with haircuts, forgetting all about the agitation he felt in those early years. The haircut process looked a bit different now. Before going to the barbershop, we would pick up French fries, so Giaci had his reward in sight. He loved having his cheering squad, his sisters, there with us and luxuriated in their praise and attention. With Giaci's increased comfort, Dad could now use his clippers without having to worry about scaring Giaci with any sharp movements. No more uneven spots or haircuts half finished; Giaci's haircuts had now become prize-worthy.

This was perhaps the first time we'd worked with and seen the power of behavioural intervention. At the time, the whole process seemed exhausting. However, as time passed, it seemed well worth it. This was another skill locked into Giaci's brain and set for life. We adapted this process to everything we could, always making sure to reward positive behaviours.

It may have taken longer to get there, but nonetheless, "we make it," as Dad always said.

TWENTY-FOUR

Such Hurtful Words

The early spring brought flowers and a renewed energy within me. I wasn't sure if I was finally getting used to our daily routines of teaching, therapy and caring for my kids and home, or if the days themselves were becoming easier. While I wished I could see more improvements in Giaci's language skills, like having a long conversation, I was happy to see he was able to follow two-step instructions. When he was asked to go pick up the toy on the floor and put it into the toybox, he could do this. When asked to find a ball and bring it to a therapist or family member, he was able to now.

Even though I still preferred to stay home, we were all getting used to attending more functions. We would go out as a family, at least once or twice a week. It was either visiting with family or friends who had a child with special needs or going out to grab a bite to eat. We were adjusting to our new normal, which meant we were not as isolated and confined to staying home. We ventured out more.

One afternoon, we planned to attend a birthday party for the son of long-time friends, Suzanne and Tim. It had been years since we saw these friends, before Giaci was born. Today was about celebrating their son who was talking and growing without any delays.

When we got to Suzanne's house, the energy in the room was cheery and joyful; it was full of laughing faces and bright smiles. However, I was uneasy because I hadn't discussed Giaci's diagnosis with anyone who was at the party. So, to avoid such a conversation, I steeled my nerves to fit in, and Actress Rita made an appearance. Beneath the surface, my attention was solely on my son and following him with my gaze.

The young children outnumbered the adults, so the room was filled with overstimulating and high-pitched voices, all interacting and playing. It was hard not to notice Giaci sitting on his own with a Dinky car, obsessing over the wheels. He sat in the corner, spinning the toy's wheels over and over again, holding it oddly close to the side of his face so he could take in a peripheral view of it.

I stood stiffly while the other parents took this time to unwind, relax, and catch up. I did not want anyone to judge my son's behaviour with the car. I knew that if I took the car away, he would have a major temper tantrum and cause an embarrassing scene. So, I left him in his world of repetition, positioning my body to shield him from others' view. The girls were not enjoying themselves either; they stayed close by to keep a watchful eye on their brother.

"I have Brian in hockey three nights a week, and Alexis has gymnastics and dance classes. Thank goodness my husband helps with hockey," Suzanne said to the crowd around her, as if her problems outweighed everyone else's in the room. What I would have given for ordinary problems like hers!

I tried to ignore the conversation, as the ease of their lives was starting to claw at me. They didn't have to deal with therapists or their child unable to express having a stomach ache. I desperately wanted to dive back into the world that used to be mine, but I simply couldn't relate. Instead, I nodded mindlessly while distracted by the painful scene in front of me. Giaci was now running back and forth on his tiptoes, flapping his hands like a bird that was ready for takeoff.

Curious eyes began to turn in his direction. A few people asked me what he was doing.

"He's a very energetic boy and loves to run. I'm thinking of signing him up for track and field." Outwardly, I shrugged it off, but inside, I was terrified that everyone would ridicule his behaviour.

From across the table, I noticed my friend Rebecca staring at Giaci with raised eyebrows. She had short dark hair and wore big gold hoop earrings that dangled. Her freckled face was stoic and cold, making my skin crawl. Why was she staring at my son? She had her own kids to take care of, so why was she scoping out *my* boy? I couldn't settle down, shifting from side to side, sensing the heavy load of judgment that was being placed on my back. I wasn't strong enough to carry it.

I wanted to sink into the ground as I saw Rebecca lean over and I heard her say something to Suzanne. All my worst fears were playing out. My son was being judged for not being "good enough" or "normal enough" or like the other kids.

Rebecca didn't even try to hide her bright coral lips, so I could see them flashing like a neon sign. I perceived her words as if she were whispering right into my ears: "He's just weird." She smirked as if her observation made her kids seem better in comparison.

My stomach was queasy, and my palms grew clammy. The appalling criticism I dreaded was surfacing. It was happening. I froze in place, not knowing how to react, so I didn't. I pretended I didn't hear her and continued to plaster a smile on my cardboard face.

She may not have even meant it in a hurtful way, but that didn't matter. It affected me like blunt trauma to the head and caused a part of me to die inside—the part that wanted to believe in the good in everyone. I hated her words and what she represented in that moment. She spewed the voice of criticism and insults. I wanted to pull my son away from this world at lightning speed and fly out of the house like Superwoman.

I kept my shoulders slumped and my eyes focused downward so I wouldn't accidentally catch anyone's gaze. I didn't dare glance around the room for fear of noticing more judging eyes. When I couldn't stand there and pretend any longer, I signalled to John that we needed to go home immediately.

"Hold him," I snapped, pushing Giaci's hand into John's. "I'm gonna get the jackets." John was perplexed by my shortness, but he still followed my instructions and stayed with Giaci while I gave the girls their jackets.

While I was trying to hurry our exit along, Giaci broke free of John's hold and ran back and forth screeching like a mouse. "Eeeeeeehhh!" Every scream stretched longer than the next, distorting time and forcing me to confront the dozens of eyes that were piercing through our world. Belittling glances circulated around the basement, communicating a knowingness that reduced me to the world's worst mother. I managed to help John scoop up Giaci and sprinted out the door with no thoughts of looking back.

* * *

On the car ride home, John noticed how upset I was, as I just couldn't settle down. My anger reverberated silently through the van. The girls were silent as soon as I buckled them into their seats. They had sensed the tension immediately once I slid the van door shut. Giaci didn't make any sounds. He was enthralled with the Dr. Seuss book that we always kept in the back seat of the van.

How could a friend say that about my son? How could anyone say such hurtful words about another person? *Weird?* How dare she! From the front passenger seat, a quasi-quiet eruption of crying burst out of me. I held my breath and bit my lip. I didn't want my children to see that I was falling apart.

John could see my face, and though he was driving, he placed his free hand on mine and asked, "What's wrong, Rita? Why are you crying?" He was completely unaware of Rebecca's comment because he'd spent the party chatting with his buddies.

I paused for a moment and took a deep breath to compose myself. The words slipped easily from my lips. "I overheard Rebecca call Giaci weird." The tears dripped off my chin. I reached into the bottom of my purse for a tissue to wipe them away. Then I mustered the strength to finish telling John what had happened.

"It was horrible, and I don't ever want to see her again!" I finished. I meant it. I hadn't seen her in years, and now I had no desire to see her anytime soon. "I don't want to have anything to do with any of them. Not her husband or their buddies. None of them!"

I had to gasp for additional air as I continued to rub the tears off my face. The kids were watching *Toy Story 2* in the back of the van. I hoped they were too preoccupied to tune in to our conversation. John paused before responding in his soft, calming voice. For once he was caught off guard by my comments.

"I didn't hear anything. Besides, it doesn't matter what anyone says. Giaci is special and we love him. That's all that matters." John always knew how to see the glass half full. He was fine with everyone knowing our son's diagnosis, but I wasn't fully there yet.

"We have a beautiful family, Rita," he continued. "Don't let Rebecca or anyone else bring you down."

I sat with my arms crossed tightly across my chest, brooding over the verbal attack on my child. Now I was angry about it.

"Should I have blasted Rebecca and embarrassed her for saying such awful things? John, I was so upset when I heard her say that about our Giaci!" I stewed in my pain.

"Let it go, Rita. Don't waste your energy. Focus your energy on our kids." John's words were always so logical. He was a master at taking the emotion out of a situation and redirecting my attention.

Breathing deeply to calm my nerves, I tried to push the event out of my head.

* * *

Our conversation ended when we arrived home, and I stomped into the house. John helped the kids out of their seatbelts and into the foyer. My internal dialogue continued to play in my head. Did I make the right choice in pretending not to hear Rebecca and walking away? Was dismissing her opinion as meaningless a safer course of action? My concern was that she was telling others what she thought and that it would soon spread like a pandemic. Everyone would know now, and maybe it was time.

Why did I care? What did it matter? Was I judging her like she was me?

With pain and fear comes defensiveness. My duty as a mother was to protect my son, but was I protecting myself more? It was clear that others were analyzing my son and my parenting, but perhaps I was projecting my own fears even more. Still, the bloodcurdling insults were what I kept hearing over and over again in my head:

"Why isn't Rita allowing him to play?"

"He must have a hearing problem. He isn't responding."

"He has a lot of energy, doesn't he?"

My heart was hardened against those casting judgments. These critics were enjoying a social life, looking pulled together and happy, and we weren't—we *weren't*.

John and I spent our days exhausted, overworked, and sleep deprived. John would often fall asleep as soon as he sat in a chair, and it was a daily struggle for me to conjure up enough energy for my students at school. The closest I ever came to doing my hair and overcoming my haggard appearance was a quick ponytail. Squeezing my eyes shut and then opening them wide to stay awake was a common occurrence.

My ego was shredded. I had no antidote for selfish pride. My fear of being negatively judged as a mother had finally come about.

As I took off the kids' jackets, I decided not to associate with Rebecca ever again.

I looked at Giaci running around the house and knew that I could not add any more pain to the heavy load I already struggled to haul. I envisioned myself carrying a tremendous number of bricks in my arms.

Each of these bricks was either a role I played or an emotion I had to deal with. There I stood in my mind's eye, juggling the sleepless nights, the financial burden, and so much more. But the heaviest bricks were the shame, guilt, and anxiety.

I had a hard enough time managing the bricks of a teacher, a sister, a daughter, a wife, and a mother of four. I was dropping bricks daily, yet still had to carry on advocating and networking, fighting depression and being a student of behavioural intervention. It was never-ending and more than any one person could sustain. From this perspective, my decision was understandable.

I disconnected from the world around me and lost my sense of pleasure. There's a clinical word for it: *anhedonia*. My heart stumbled over its own rhythm because nothing was fulfilling. I didn't care anymore. For my own well-being, I didn't give those critics any more headspace.

You could care about people like Rebecca and still choose to not interact with them. You could miss that person every day and still be glad they were no longer complicating your life or distracting your focus. I realized that what anyone thought of my son *shouldn't* matter. *My* thoughts of him were what had value, and I couldn't have anyone tainting my focus and my opinion of my child.

TWENTY-FIVE

The Old-School Mentality

Sunday after Sunday I would venture out with the kids and go to church. This Sunday, I hoped I might be able to get through a complete Mass at church with all four of them.

Our parish was the Italian church that sat in the very centre of the Italian community, where John and I had made many sacraments. Built in 1939, it was an old Roman Catholic Church for the Italian immigrant community, and it had now grown to include two or three generations of families. It was meant to preserve the cultural and religious beliefs of all the Italians in the area, and it gave us all a sense of tradition and community. The churchgoers were mainly first-generation Italian immigrants who spoke the dialects of their hometowns, which were sometimes difficult to understand.

When the morning came, I made sure to dress the kids and myself in our Sunday best.

I grew up knowing that there was an unwritten expectation to dress up for church; it was one of those "proper etiquette" rules that I was raised with. We were expected to show a higher level of respect for God through how we presented ourselves, both physically and spiritually.

I made sure the girls' hair was coiffed with braids and cute little bow-shaped hair clips. They wore floral-print dresses; Lauren's was a fit-and-flare style, while the twins wore the same style dress but in different colours. Carolina was always in pink, and Maria was always in blue. Their girly dresses were trimmed with either a little lace or ribbon, just like mine had been as a child. Giaci was decked out in his adorable little dress pants and a dress shirt that never stayed tucked in, no matter how hard I tried. On the outside, we were presentable, but what it took to get there was another story. Beneath the polished surface were hours of making sure no one got dirty or wrecked their hair before showtime.

Since there were four children to prepare, by the time I had Giaci and Lauren dressed and coiffed, Carolina and Maria had gotten into the cupboard and were eating chocolate chip cookies. They sat with their dresses sprawled around them and wore a lip tint of chocolate around their grins. When I caught them, I ran their hands and mouths beneath the faucet. I had no time to fix their hair, which was undone and sticking to their cheeks and the napes of their necks from running around.

I should have accepted the reality that we would never show up to church looking like a perfectly polished family and just grab the bag I'd prepared for the kids. It was filled with early reader books and fidget toys to entertain them during Mass. We weren't perfect, but at least we would make it.

Every week, the kids and I tried to get through the entire church service, which was difficult for Giaci since he was expected to sit noiselessly for almost an hour. This was a difficult task for many adults, but for Giaci it was like climbing Mount Everest without water. He would begin vibrating his voice, as if trying to sing along, and he couldn't sit still.

The old-school Italian mentality is that children should be seen and not heard, and it remained true in this particular community.

That's what finally broke me. We entered and found our seats, once again, with all eyes on us. I averted my gaze to avoid eye contact. I had already decided not to care what others thought and instead protected Giaci as the incense filled the air. Between the creaking wooden pews and foggy atmosphere, he was already fidgety. I wouldn't add to his discomfort with my own tension.

On this day, as the priest walked from the back of the church toward the altar, I noticed his wrinkled finger lift to his lips, his dreary eyes locked on our family. His procession took small steps behind him, mimicking his stuffy attitude toward us. As if it were their sworn duty, the rest of the flock fell in line with their eyes, casting glares and disappointment in our direction because they knew from past church ceremonies that Giaci would make noise and interrupt the Mass. I snapped. I didn't have to sit through this, and neither did my children. With a loud rustle—one that could be made only by my four children—I stormed us out and didn't look back.

* * *

As soon as John got home, he got an earful.

"And we've been going there our whole lives! The nerve of those people, John. As if *their* children didn't make noise." I sat on the edge of our bed, muttering and complaining.

John's eyes widened, as if he'd suddenly had an idea. "Why don't you start going to St. Mary's Catholic church near our new house?" He was close to completing another custom build, so we would be moving again soon.

"But..." I paused, wondering what our parents would think about our leaving the Italian church. "It's our tradition." Even as I said it, it didn't feel right anymore. It didn't feel like the place where I'd celebrated so many Holy Sacraments. My desire to maintain our Catholic religion remained, and it was important to us to pass that on to our children.

"We can make new traditions," John suggested. "This is our family, and we make our own rules."

He was right. What was keeping me tied to a church where I felt no one wanted us? Between Rebecca and now our old church, it felt like we were shedding everything and everyone from our old lives. Just the thought of it left me feeling lighter, and I knew that I had to act on that gut feeling.

* * *

The following week, I took John's advice, and we started attending Mass at the new Catholic church. This church was more modern-looking, with straight lines, fewer statues, and minimal stained-glass windows. It had a much simpler feel than our old, traditional church.

I parked the van, took a deep breath and called out to God for the first time in months.

Please accept us. Please let my children in, I practically begged. I knew that if this church didn't work either, I wouldn't make them go anymore. I was finished with trying to force people into our lives who didn't want us.

One by one, I helped the kids out of the van. Giaci was always the last one out due to my fear that he would run away. As I always did, I clenched his hand so he was unable to leave my side, and we walked toward the church together. Surrounded by our family, we took one small step after another into the church.

As we entered, the organ played, and the congregation smiled. The casual aura felt good, yet I trembled inside. Was it safe to enjoy this moment? They didn't know us yet.

The grey-haired priest stood at the back of the church greeting people as they entered. We tried to scurry past him to go unnoticed, but he spotted us. I glanced over at him and nodded with a timid smile, clinging to my children. He approached and welcomed us with a smile. "Who do we have here?" he asked, looking down at my entire world.

Lauren gave a brief "hello," and Carolina held up her little hand with a teeny wave. Maria smiled and hid herself behind my blue-and-white-striped skirt. All three displayed their usual reactions, but Giaci wouldn't divert his gaze even for a moment. I felt the need to explain.

"Father, my son has autism," I said, still not fully comfortable declaring his diagnosis out loud. "I'd like to apologize in advance if he gets loud during the Mass. It can be challenging for him to sit still, and he does get overstimulated at times."

His expression shifted from delighted to surprised.

He nodded and placed both of his pale hands on Giaci's head. Giaci froze as the priest's hands cupped his head. "No need to apologize, my dear. We are in God's house, and not only are we all welcomed, but we are all embraced with open arms, especially the special ones." He smiled at me just as the musical crescendo echoed through the pews. It swelled around my shoulders like a fleece shawl welcoming me home. I hadn't felt so at ease in a long time. It was uplifting to feel that spiritual embrace again.

I was still holding Giaci by the hand, and we all paused for a moment, taking in every musical note. When the priest released him and moved on to greet the next family, I guided my children into our new sanctuary.

We positioned ourselves in the last pew, which was our preferred spot in case we needed to make a quick getaway. The angelic sounds of the choir filled our ears, and we watched as the priest walked toward the altar.

I replayed the priest's words in my mind, *especially the special ones*, feeling comfort and harmony and finding beauty in his acceptance. I realized that this could be our life if we would simply open ourselves up to others rather than continue to hide away. During silent prayer, the kids maintained their composure, which allowed me to tap into my connection with God once again. Suddenly, a sense of knowing came over me, as if God were signalling to my heart to open itself up. I'd felt this only a few times before in my life. When I let God in, I realized it had been in me to do so this entire time. I had been the one afraid to let Him in and to see Him within my son. I had been afraid to let anyone in to see the real Giaci.

This truth gripped at my throat. *I* had been the one keeping us prisoner within our own home, not autism.

At the end of my meditation, I looked up at the priest, who was looking our way with love and acceptance. I finally felt God's—and my own—love. I looked over at my squirming children, their eyes fluttering in their own sort of prayer, and I knew no matter what changed around us, we'd always have each other.

TWENTY-SIX

Let Go and Trust God

At first it was hard to let go of the long-standing traditions that tied us to our old parish. The unspoken rule growing up had been to stay loyal to our Italian roots and encourage this devotion in the next generation.

We were bound to that church by the big moments in our lives, like my First Communion. My mother had created my white lace dress especially for this occasion. The Italian church was packed to the brim with smiling families as they watched their children receive this sacrament. It didn't matter if it was your biological child or not; the entire community celebrated their honorary children going through this holy rite of passage together.

In photos, you didn't see just immediate family filling the dining hall for the ceremony. Relatives from near and far, no matter how distantly related, filled the corners of the room. Each scene played out in my mind: the endless buffet of food, the kisses pressed on cheeks, the polkas and tarantellas danced until our feet blistered.

Letting go of the Italian church was about more than letting go of a space. It had been a part of my and John's cultural upbringing. But if I wanted my kids to have any relationship with God, the new church, St. Mary's, would be the answer. That our kids kept our faith was more important to me than the place that kept it for them.

It felt as if God had been trying to teach me a lesson about being in charge of our own lives and deciding what and who was best for our family. God was also whispering to me, encouraging me to let go of judgment. Before, I couldn't allow myself to hear the whisper. Now, the whisper was turning into a roar that I could no longer ignore.

God spoke through my children.

"Mommy, I like going to church! People are nice," Maria said with her almost-four-year-old innocence as we got ready for another Sunday at St. Mary's Church. Her intuitive mind was aware of her surroundings, much like Lauren's.

"That's good, honey. I'm glad," I said with a gentle caress under her chin.

Stepping through these new doors each week gave me a feeling of total acceptance, which I had rarely experienced over the last five years. The environment of calm resonated with the kids too—even Giaci, who walked quietly beside his sisters as we took our seats. Other kids would run off to Sunday school, leaving their parents to pray, but I couldn't leave Giaci with just anyone, no matter how much progress we'd made. I also needed the girls to stay with me to model good listening for Giaci.

Giaci was now able to imitate behaviours during Mass, and I would interject brief moments of learning so he would be able to participate alongside us. Using hand-over-hand techniques, I would guide his hand to make the sign of the cross. First, we touched his forehead with our fingers, and he repeated "In the name of the Father." Then, we moved down to his chest with "and of the Son." My hand steered his from his left shoulder to his right to finish with "and of the Holy Spirit, amen." To end this sacramental action, I manoeuvred his little hands together in prayer.

Every week he made progress with these actions, one step at a time, until he was able to do them independently. We reinforced him with smiles and praise, which motivated him and kept him striving for more. Once the behaviour was reinforced, it would stay with Giaci week after week.

The girls were gleeful to see their brother access these skills and participate throughout the Mass. If he forgot any movements, they coached him along. Their little hands glided over his as they all began creating a new faith for themselves. It was a faith in God, but also a faith in each other, a faith that told them they'd always be able to count on one another. Pride echoed through all of us as Giaci's learning was a team effort, and we all shared in his successes.

"Giaci can do anything, as long as we teach him, right, Mommy?" Carolina asked one Sunday as Giaci settled calmly into the pew.

"Yes, that's right, honey, as long as we are patient with him," I whispered.

I hadn't realized how much of my teaching would rub off on the girls, or how much responsibility they would take on for their brother. I tried not to force them into caring for their brother; instead, I invited them to help him with me. Making them a part of this process solidified their tight-knit sibling bond.

A sense of peace washed over me as the hymn began, and with a sense of calm, I was able to imagine them taking my place. I knew this would happen one day, and seeing them forge a strong connection early on gave me the strength to keep going.

When the hymn ended, I sang a final "amen," thanking God for these gifts before exchanging the gesture of peace with our new extended family. Again, I guided Giaci through this sensory experience with a hand-over-hand technique. We would shake friendly parishioners' hands, and they smiled in delight at the progress he showed week after week. The support we received was uplifting, and soon, when gestured to at the appropriate time, Giaci would shake hands independently and say, "Peace be with you." Parishioners cheered him on, showing big smiles and nods of approval.

As we sat again, we waited for the priest to approach the altar to conclude the Mass. He raised his arms upward to quiet the choir before he spoke. The entire congregation was silent when a powerful roar erupted from my son's backside and onto the pew. The entire wooden pew vibrated, giving us a thunderous shake. Giaci sat more comfortably in his spot now, undisturbed by his addition to the service. Meanwhile, all three of my daughters sank down in their spots; their stunned eyes bulged from their flushed faces.

Their heads pivoted immediately, turning their beet-red faces to me, as if I could rectify the situation. Six eyes blazed into me, as if this were the most embarrassing moment the girls could ever possibly experience.

"Just look forward at the priest and pretend you didn't hear it," I whispered through the side of my mouth.

They complied, not knowing what else to do. The parishioners around us didn't react either, knowing the extent of our embarrassment. They knew where the sound came from, but they also knew that we couldn't control my little man's natural body.

Giaci had no social inhibitions and did not understand that his loud fart was socially inappropriate. It didn't faze him in the least.

The girls continued to gaze at the priest, but I could tell by the tension in their foreheads that they just wanted to bolt out of there. I couldn't help but let out a little giggle, which invited the girls to let theirs out too. What else could we have done, short of putting a cork in it? I was out of solutions; teaching Giaci to hold in a fart was impossible. He would fart at home, or at the grandparents' houses, but farting at a silent moment in church with about 100 people hearing it, as it echoed through the high ceiling, was a different experience. So, we all giggled under our breath while we kept our heads down for the final prayer.

Once we were a few feet away from the church, Maria finally burst. "How embarrassing! Giaci farted so loud!"

Carolina slapped her knee as she giggled, and we all hooted with laughter, sharing the funny side of their most embarrassing moment. Lauren let out a boisterous, contagious laugh.

As young as the girls were, they modelled mature behaviour on an ongoing basis. Having a brother with special needs made them mature earlier than other siblings might have. The girls were raised knowing that Giaci's condition required the whole family to work together to help him. They embraced it and showed tremendous love for him in a beautiful way by not resenting him for any of it. They understood that one member of the family impacts everyone and that the strengths they had could help their brother. They understood devotion for the family unit.

TWENTY-SEVEN

An Italian-Style Field Trip

After our hilarious Sunday service, we arrived home just as the phone rang.

It was Mom calling to tell me about a religious retreat organized by the Italian church. "There is a religious retreat, and I'd like you and Giaci to come," Mom said in Italian. She wanted me to bring Giaci because she felt that a special blessing would help him recover from his delays.

"Uh, I really don't want to go," I said, turned off by the idea of a daylong retreat with the older generation of parishioners.

If she heard the hesitation in my voice, she didn't acknowledge it.

"For Giaci," she said, tempting me the only way she knew how. "You, me, and your in-laws—we all go."

I could have made a fuss and declined, but sometimes with family it's easier to give in and say yes.

It wasn't until that moment that I realized how much my parents and in-laws were struggling with Giaci's diagnosis. When I told them that Giaci had "special needs," they understood it as him being delayed. Any explicit discussion of autism had never actually happened because the complexity of autism was difficult for them to comprehend fully. Other family members and friends knew about Giaci's autism, yet there wasn't much discussion of it. Regardless, they understood Giaci was "special," and in their minds, praying to God would help him catch up.

The weather was bright and warm on the day we left for the retreat, a sign of good luck for our travels and for the grandparents' mission to pray for a cure for their grandson. The bus to the Basilica and National

Shrine of Our Lady of Consolation in Carey, a village in northwestern Ohio, was full. This so-called "retreat" felt more like an Italian field trip, one to which my parents and in-laws arrived armed with rosaries in hand and snacks in their bags.

The bus soon began to absorb the scents of Italian-style cured meats. Wafts of prosciutto, salami, and soppressata seeped into the seats. Homemade biscotti, cheeses, and olives completed the spread, as "snacks" were really a full meal for Italians. Our culture's deep connection to food floated from one seat to the next, and it subsided only to substitute the smell of food for that of bitter espresso steaming up the windows. Women had thermoses filled with the concentrate and were passing them around like kids hiding a flask at a school dance.

Giaci and I were the youngest passengers by far, and we were surrounded by an entire generation of Italian immigrants. A sigh of relief washed over me when I realized that the two-hour bus ride would be air conditioned; if it were otherwise, all celebration would have been replaced by rhythmic cursing in every Italian dialect.

Each section of the bus was divided like a map of Italy; everyone sat with others from their region. The southern Sicilians sat together speaking in their dialect, while the northern Italians sat on the other end of the bus speaking among themselves in *their* distinct dialect. I could only understand the southerners because that is the dialect I was raised speaking. Giaci wasn't bothered by the loud chatter on the bus because he was being fed by all the nonnas.

"*Cu fu?*" said one *paesano* to another as they gossiped wondering, "Who did it?" to other fellow countrymen. I wasn't inclined to eavesdrop; all I took away from the conversation was that "what that person did was a mystery." It was an Italian version of the "who's on first" script by Abbott and Costello.

I kept Giaci occupied on the bus with snacks and videos until we arrived at the sanctuary, where every Italian woman took out a little plastic water container that had a small gold cross dangling from its front. They were going to fill these containers with holy water blessed by the clergymen. Holy water is used to bless a person or repel evil. It was the weapon of choice for Italian mothers and nonnas.

One by one we disembarked from the boisterous bus. As each person exited the bus, they made the sign of the cross, kissing their finger to seal their genuine love for and belief in the Lord. I held Giaci tightly, as I always did, afraid of him tearing away from my grip and running off.

Standing off to the side, waiting for my in-laws and parents to get off the bus, I reflected on why I had agreed to come. There is no cure for autism; this was not going to take Giaci's autism away. But to appease his grandparents, I had come along because it was what *they* needed to believe. They were here to pray the autism away, and I had to admit that there was—and always would be—a little piece of me that still hoped for such a miracle.

When the grandparents got off the bus, they walked over to us and kissed Giaci on the head. They were doing this for him, and Giaci didn't understand why we were there, so who was I to deny them this comfort?

We all proceeded to the shrine of the Virgin Mary. As we walked, I noticed the crumbling brick and stone on the outside of this old, weathered church. I was in awe of the sculpted detail in the arches of the ceiling and the hand-painted images of the Lord and saints on the walls. The flickering flames of the vigil candles represented faith and prayers, each paying homage to the Blessed Mother Mary. The smell of burning wax sank into our pores.

As we approached, I could see that every person kissed their first two fingers and then touched the statue of La Madonna and the other statues of saints. Everyone was reserved, displaying their spiritual respect. Women retrieved their rosaries, holding each bead ever so gently as they chanted prayers over and over again. My mom and mother-in-law, after kissing the feet of the Madonna statue, touched Giaci on the head, as if

Mother Mary's magical powers would be transferred to my son. Giaci barely flinched at their touch; he was behaving extremely well given all the walking and silent time. His belly was full, so he seemed satisfied.

To most it would have seemed like an exorcism ceremony, but to me it was a sign of their faith, which they believed would help their grandson. Their prayers were so intense and passionate. Raw emotion was evident on the women's faces. They believed that God and the Blessed Mother Mary would provide sublime intervention. They willed it through their spiritual beliefs, reminding me of the early days when I also tried to pray Giaci's autism away. This was how they coped with Giaci's disability. They felt that this was their strongest contribution to him.

Lined up like sheep following a shepherd in the fields, we formed a procession line, walking at a leisurely pace behind La Madonna.

Many of the older men wore their *coppola* hats, and most women wore dress pants and blouses, clutching their leather purses as they walked in an orderly fashion. Everyone prayed as we marched obediently behind the statue that was held above our heads. They prayed, calling on all the saints, angels, and dearly departed to help with their specific religious requests. They prayed in such a powerful way that it caused my throat to ache and brought tears to my eyes. I had to step out of the procession to compose myself.

For the first time all day, Giaci was growing bored and tired and was starting to fuss. I took him to the bathroom in the basement of the church to gather my thoughts and to give him a break. I took a deep breath as I once again came face-to-face with the new Rita in the mirror. I had spent so many days looking her in the eye and begging her to go back to normal. I thought that maybe by finding the normalcy in myself, I'd be able to find some normalcy for Giaci as well. This new Rita had colour back in her cheeks and her hair was combed to the side, slightly above her mascaraed eyes. My reflection bounced back at me like the shine of water waves.

Now, being there with all the praying grandparents, I realized that they were just as desperate—if not more so—to help him as I was. Seeing how they gazed at their grandson with such anguish and pain in their eyes, I realized that I wouldn't have been so alone in my desperation and loss if I had shared it with them sooner. This was an important lesson I wish I'd learned earlier. The grandparents were experiencing the loss too, though on a different level, as observers. They hadn't struggled with the daily realities of autism, hadn't stayed up with him for days at a time, struggling to balance all other aspects of their lives while endlessly trying to get help for him.

My shoulders began to shake as I clutched the sides of the bathroom sink. Giaci stood by my side for a few minutes, but then began running around the locked bathroom. Watching his grandparents yearn for the same thing I had yearned for—for years—only solidified our lifelong reality. This wasn't going away, no matter how hard we prayed or begged God.

There were so many times when my parents tried to reassure me, as if they'd seen Giaci's behaviour before in other children.

"He gonna be okay," Dad said in his broken English as he gently patted my shoulder. "When he go through *lo sviluppo*, he gonna be okay. I know." He believed that once my son reached puberty, he would self-correct and catch up to typically developing children.

It was hard to hear. For a time, part of me hoped this was true, but now, with Giaci being almost six years old, I knew it just wasn't the case. There was no outgrowing autism.

Only recently, I had begun to glimpse the life we could have—my girls, Giaci, John and I—and it was beautiful. We were so affectionate with each other, always hugging and saying, "I love you." Praising each other constantly was our new norm. No more negativity or unrealistic expectations. Our family was growing stronger, and there had been more and more wonderful and easy days. I couldn't spend any more of my time trying to will away our challenges, not when there were bigger things to focus on. I had to enjoy my life with my kids and my husband.

In the church bathroom, I made a small sign of the cross, thanking God for another realization.

I would let the grandparents pray for their miracle, but I knew that we were moving toward the next phase in our lives. No matter what was ahead, we could handle it. We were built for it by the very people waiting outside.

Stitched into our beings were the strength, perseverance, and faith of our parents. And that was more than enough.

PART THREE

Transformation

TWENTY-EIGHT

Reaching Out

For almost a year, I carried around a small piece of paper in my wallet. It was folded twice, making it even smaller than it needed to be. On that piece of paper were the letters *AO* and a phone number. AO stood for Autism Ontario, and the phone number was to our local chapter.

Autism Ontario is a provincial organization that aims to promote "acceptance of and opportunities for" individuals on the autism spectrum. The organization has chapters across the province, run by families who volunteer their time to help others in their community. Autism Ontario information appeared again and again in my various internet searches. I had written down the phone number thinking I would call this organization, only to lose my nerve every time. Fear of the unknown always held me back.

Each time I clutched that little piece of paper, my hands shook. Even though I was making progress in accepting Giaci's diagnosis, calling this number would be like a public broadcast. But I was tired of holding back: I needed to just do it. And so, one day, I gathered my thoughts, lowered my shield, and finally dialed the number.

As the phone rang, I thought about the questions the person on the other end of the line might ask: *What do you need? What do you need help with?* The only word that resonated through my mind with each ring was *everything*. We needed everything.

"Hello! Autism Ontario. How can I help you?" a cheerful female voice said from the other end. She sounded eager to help, not like the government monotone I'd experienced so many times before.

My voice got caught for a moment before letting go. "Ah, yes, hello. I'm just wondering what type of services you offer families," I started slowly.

"We're a not-for-profit organization of volunteers like me who make themselves available to families. It all depends on what the family members need! Families join our parent or sibling groups because they want to talk to others who are going through similar autism experiences."

Her explanation slipped out with ease, as if she genuinely believed in the place she volunteered at. That flicker of a sense of home grew brighter within me as she continued explaining the Autism Ontario space. "We also have a lending library filled with resources, books, and videos for families to borrow for their kids."

"Wow, that's nice!" My enthusiasm prevented a more intelligent response.

"It sure is! What can I help you with?"

Everything.

I paused, trying to figure out how to word it. In the meantime, I decided to simply learn more. "Who am I speaking with? You said you were a volunteer, but in what capacity?"

"My name is Kyla, and I am a mother of a child with autism. I am currently the vice president of this chapter. Are you a professional in the field of autism, or do you have a child with autism?"

In the past, this question would have stunned me. Old habits almost forced the phone down, but this was what we needed. Giaci and I both needed a community.

"I'm an educator," I said, "and my son was diagnosed at three years old." I cleared my throat. "And um...I have three daughters." I blinked twice as I took another breath.

Her voice perked up with motherly knowing.

"Having a child with autism is hard to deal with. Just getting a diagnosis is difficult. You may not know what to do or say, but our organization is here for you whenever you're ready."

Relief touched parts of me that had been tense for years.

She continued. "You may want to get involved as well. Volunteering has been very fulfilling for me. The most important advice I can give you is to talk with other parents who are in a similar situation."

This call wasn't as uncomfortable as I'd imagined it would be. Common ground connected us.

"If there's anything I can do to help you," she added, "call me back anytime. Remember, I've been in your shoes too. We're in this together."

"Okay, thank you."

Even after Kyla hung up, her words stayed with me. For so long, I hadn't felt like I was in this with anyone, and here was this stranger—this other mom—who was easier to talk to than my own friends.

I made a habit of calling back week after week.

One time Kyla and I spoke for longer than usual, and she informed me of the parent meeting dates and when the upcoming information nights were.

She must have sensed my apprehension because she continued to repeat how important it was to connect with others. "We'd really love to have you! Just try. Come out to one of our meetings."

"I'll do my best," I said, writing down the same information for the fourth time. I couldn't let this become like the Autism Ontario number I carried in my wallet for a year. That initial call had turned out better than I'd expected, so maybe I could muster the courage for an in-person meeting. "No, really. I will try to make it," I repeated. I had to at least try, for Giaci's sake.

Before long I was attending as many meetings as I possibly could, empowered by the information I was taking in. I met new people and made connections, and with each visit I learned something new that helped Giaci and our family.

With each visit there was an awakening; the unknown was becoming known, and here I was, still standing. Nothing pushed me to the ground. Thanks to the information other parents shared, my awareness of what autism was expanded. We all shared stories. I heard what other parents were doing for their children with autism. I realized that other parents were struggling with the same issues that my family struggled with, such as sleepless nights, a lack of focus, lack of social interactions and delayed social and language skills.

At one meeting, five mothers and two fathers attended. Every one of us had a son with autism. Since autism is more common in boys, this wasn't surprising. The discussion topic that night was "What to do about your picky eater." We brainstormed strategies and exchanged recipes.

One dad, named Ivan, shared that his son would stop eating altogether until he got exactly what he wanted. He could go days without eating.

"My wife and I have tried everything, but he just wants to eat French fries. So I just give it to him. It's easier, and we can't let him starve. He has to eat!"

Another mother named Samantha brought a suggestion to the table. "I add puréed vegetables to foods my son eats. He doesn't even know they're in there. It's working for now, so maybe you could try that?"

Ivan smiled back with thanks. We all appreciated the generous and empathetic feedback and understanding we received at these meetings. It was like we were veterans exchanging war stories, each knowing the battles the others had been through. There is something to be said about connecting with others who have had similar experiences in life. It's connecting at a deeper level.

After hearing Samantha and Ivan's stories, I realized that my approach to getting my son to eat was a little different. In both examples, the child was in control. Their sons were either getting what they wanted, or they were being tricked into compliance.

"May I share?" I spoke up for the first time, unsure if anyone would be interested in or responsive to my technique. When everyone nodded, I began telling them about my "First, one bite of broccoli" technique. "It works with any vegetable or other undesired foods, and you reward them with a bite of desired food, like French fries." I continued to explain how the undesired food is introduced slowly and progressively increased. "Then, in time, I tell him that he has to take two bites before I give him the chips he wants." This technique had been working thus far for me because I didn't give him any other option and he still felt like he was winning the food battle.

The other parents' initial response was a few moments of silence as they took in my suggestion. It was a simple concept, but clearly no one had thought of it or even attempted it.

Ivan spoke first. "That would never work with my son."

Samantha said, "I'm gonna try it. I'll let you know how it goes!"

Sharing my experiences and hearing about theirs was creating a new-found community that gave me a sense of belonging. It was a support system that filled a void I had been lost in. I realized how important it was to reach out for support and to make the most of it. Another life lesson learned.

* * *

On my way out of the meeting that night, I ran into another mom, Janice. Her son, Timothy, was about the same age as Giaci, and we bonded over a shared vision for our boys.

"Timothy will say 'hello,' but that's about it right now," Janice told me as we walked down the corridor.

"It's hard that we can't have a full conversation with them, isn't it?" I echoed. "We're still working on functional language skills. It's my dream to have a conversation with Giaci."

My words came so easily in this space, with these people. I'd resisted this help for so long and ached knowing what it would have been like to have had this support from the start. At least I had it now.

I touched Janice's shoulder with understanding before we parted ways. This was the beginning of a strong kinship between Janice and me. We were two moms at the starting line on the track that is autism. The infamous timer was set, and we were ready, hoping for a steady incline on the trajectory of our sons' development and growth.

TWENTY-NINE

Two Mothers on a Mission

Soon, Janice and I were touching base almost every day. Since we were working toward the same goal, we shared the titles of books we were reading on autism, health, and wellness, and we talked at length about our sons' obsessions with certain foods and their overall nutrition. When we couldn't attend meetings, we would chat over the phone just to share how our days were going.

"Rita, you're not going to believe what happened today," Janice said one day over the phone. I'd never heard her so excited. "I looked up Dr. Rimland and found his phone number!" Dr. Bernard Rimland was the coauthor, with William Shaw, of a book we'd both recently read called *Biological Treatments for Autism and PDD*. Rimland was credited with debunking the "refrigerator mother" theory—that autism came from emotionally cold mothers. While instrumental to revolutionizing modern autism medicine, Bernard Rimland's stance on the causality between vaccines and autism has since been disproven. At that time, his book was a comprehensive and easy-to-read guide to the most current research and medical therapies for autism and PDD. However, he incorrectly led many parents to believe that autism was caused by vaccines. His approach to "curing" autism, which he called Defeat Autism Now! (DAN!), led many to undertake risky and expensive treatments.

I was one of them with regards to the expensive treatment. Many parents felt that the DAN! Protocol (founded in 1995) "cured" their children, but there was virtually no research evidence that supported this.

I was only listening to what I wanted to hear. Janice was doing the same. We were enthralled by how his research was offering hope for a "cure."

We read about leaky gut syndrome, a digestive condition that affects the lining of the intestines. It explained how the gaps in the intestinal walls allow bacteria and other toxins to pass into the bloodstream. As a result, the body is unable to make the normal connections with the brain, hence the gut/brain disconnection. Could this be what our sons had?

"So? Did you call him?" I said. I couldn't believe that she'd spoken to a person who could provide a vital missing piece of the puzzle, or so I thought.

"I had to! And he picked up! We discussed biological treatments and how to help our sons," she gushed as if she'd just called a celebrity. "He gave me some really great advice and told me to connect with Dr. Krone next. Rita, I Googled her, and I think our boys will improve once their bodies are nourished properly."

I joined her in this impossible high. She and I both wanted to believe that this was the answer we had been searching for.

Feeding off her excitement, I was compelled to embrace this supposed miraculous remedy. My heart yearned for a cure, but my brain was fully aware that there was no cure for autism. Still, the energy that hit me after our conversation ignited my next round of internet searches. I took to the web to find Dr. Krone and learned that she was not a medical doctor but had a doctorate in nutrition, specializing in body chemistry. She was the director of the Neuro-Molecular Foundation in Albany, New York, and her research pointed to the importance of helping the body cure itself by balancing its chemistry through bio-metabolic intervention. She'd even shown success with children with autism, specifically.

I was intrigued and couldn't wait to call Janice back to discuss what I'd read.

"Janice, everything sounds really promising. I think we have to connect with this doctor."

"Let's call her together tomorrow. I can come over in the morning!"

After hanging up, I filled John in on everything; he was intrigued by the possibilities and supported the idea of Janice and me travelling to New York with our boys to meet Dr. Krone. The prospects of a causal relationship between balancing our son's body chemistry and seeing an improvement in speech and social skills were a fascinating new direction.

Prior to our trip, Dr. Krone emailed some paperwork for us to fill out and suggested getting bloodwork done before meeting in person.

The paperwork contained many questions about eating habits. Giaci loved eating McDonald's French fries, cereal, and pasta. Timothy's fixations were on Goldfish crackers and chips. Even though I could convince Giaci to eat fruits and vegetables, it still wasn't an optimal health regimen. Janice had simply given into Timothy's tendencies and allowed him to eat whatever he wanted; otherwise, he wouldn't eat at all. He would protest by not eating for days unless he was given what he wanted.

From what I had read, up to three-quarters of families with children who have autism try alternative therapies. We were about to be included in those statistics.

* * *

Once we'd booked our flights, car rental, and accommodations, we were all set to go see Dr. Krone.

John and I agreed that it would be best if just Giaci and I went so John could work and take care of the girls. I made sure to let my mother and mother-in-law know that I was taking Giaci to see a "special doctor" in New York. Mom was ready and willing to give support.

"You wanna me to come with you?" she boomed over the phone. I could hear shuffling in the background as if she were already packing her bags.

"No, that's okay, Ma. I'm going with another mom and her son," I answered.

"Oh, okay, as long as you no go alone!" She didn't ask any further questions about the trip, instead changing the subject by asking me what I was preparing for dinner.

We were going to be away for three days, and I wanted to make sure Giaci saw his grandparents before we left. So, the day before we left, I went over to their houses to say goodbye.

Dad embraced Giaci with a manly squeeze. Mom placed her hands on his beautiful round head. I could hear her mumbling the "Our Father" prayer under her breath. After they loaded us up with snacks and pasta for Giaci, we made our way to the second set of grandparents. I could see the sadness in Mom's eyes as I drove off.

Nonno Giacinto greeted Giaci similarly by covering the entire top of his head with his thick hands and tapping him gently. Giaci didn't move as he was comforted by the deep-pressure tapping coming from above. Nonna Carolina grabbed the sides of his face, squeezing aggressively, and planted a firm kiss on his cheek. She then gave us her warning of concern:

"*Sta attento.*"

She wagged her finger at us to be mindful. We'd never travelled this far on our own, and even though they understood my independence, her wary look told me that she wished John was coming along.

As I drove away down their long cement driveway, in the corner of my eye I could see my mother-in-law sending us off with the sign of the cross.

* * *

At the airport, Giaci and I connected with Janice and Timothy, though they weren't alone. Janice's cousin Hope greeted us with butterscotch eyes that sweetened the stress we all felt. Janice and Hope were kindred spirits, finishing each other's sentences and anticipating each other's needs.

"We need to go to the bathroom before we board. Can you grab the—"

"Bags and purses? Got 'em." Hope jumped to the rescue. I didn't know her well, but I was already delighted to have her with us.

The plane ride went smoothly, and even though it was his first trip, Giaci didn't seem fazed at all by the multiple alterations to his day. Once we arrived in New York, we rented a minivan. I drove while Janice dictated directions from the passenger seat and Hope minded the boys in the back. Giaci was securely belted into the seat behind me, so I had a clear view of him in the rear-view mirror, playing with his VTech electronic laptop and Leapfrog toys—with crackers nearby.

While I drove, I constantly tried to engage Giaci. I was still relentless about using every second for learning.

"Hi, Giaci!" I said. "Mommy loves you, buddy."

He would answer my call with "Hi, Mommy. More snacks!" and then go back to playing his spelling game, which responded in a robotic female voice. "Spell *cat*, C-A-T," she would say mechanically. Then, as his little fingers pressed the letters, she would congratulate him. When she echoed "Nice job!" Giaci would glance up at me and then continue to play.

"We're almost there," Janice said. "Turn right here. The building up ahead is where we need to go."

I parked the van, quickly jumped out, and opened the back sliding door to retrieve Giaci, who was still preoccupied with his toy computer. My breathing deepened in rapid anticipation of our first encounter with Dr. Krone.

"Come on, Giaci! We're going to see Dr. Krone," I said, as if he could understand everything I was saying. Giaci cast a brief glance at me as I took his seatbelt off.

"Ready, set, go, buddy!" I often tried to keep him interested in what we did by injecting fun little games into basic activities, such as getting out of the van. "On the count of three, you gotta jump into Mommy's arms." I clapped my hands and proceeded with our one-way conversation.

"Ready? One," I said and paused, waiting for his eyes to connect with mine.

"T-w-o…". I stretched that word out longer to give him extra time to react.

"Three!" My voice went higher, as it was the culmination of my game to have him make his move.

"Jump! Jump, Giaci, go!" I waited, anticipating his jump into my outstretched arms. Giaci caught sight of me, smiled, and jumped into my arms. As he wrapped his skinny little arms around my neck, our connection surrounded me like a soft blanket. My son's embrace gave me such inner warmth and calm. It brought my heart rate back down to a regular beat. He gave me the strength to walk toward the unknown.

Out of the corner of my eye, I saw Janice watching us with interest. She looked so tired. I thought back over our trip: Janice and Timothy hadn't engaged much at all the entire time. She did everything for him. She spoke for him and about him. I was afraid she had lost the motivation to push her son. When a child doesn't respond and it goes on and on, it can be disheartening. Janice took off Timothy's seatbelt, scooped him out of the car seat carefully, grabbed his hand, and tried to lead him toward the building. He was so resistant; it was like she was pulling him. Hope picked up the snack and toy bags and, without saying a word, walked behind them.

As the five of us moved toward Dr. Krone's office, my anxiety came on full force. It was like a brisk day that sent a chill up my spine, or was it just the fear of the unknown? New York weather was comparable to home, but New York didn't look like home. The building was new, and it looked empty. There weren't many cars in the parking lot, just our van and three other vehicles. Perhaps it was because this was a special weekend meeting arranged just for us. I bit my lip, hoping this wasn't all for nothing.

My grip on Giaci was stronger than ever; I didn't dare lose sight of him in this foreign place. When we reached the office waiting room, my grip didn't loosen, especially since Janice was struggling to keep Timothy calm. He was running around, trying to escape her grip, and crying all the while.

Unable to control Timothy, Janice grabbed him and placed him on her lap in an attempt to stop him from running in circles. Physically restricting his movement was possible because Timothy was little, and she was stronger. But what would happen when our boys got bigger and stronger? Over time, holding him or forcing him to do something would become impossible. As difficult as it was to imagine now, the reality was that our boys would turn into men, and we would weaken with age. These were important factors that we needed to consider. My goal was to teach at all times; my constant motivating mantra was "Early intervention is key," and teaching was in my blood.

Janice must have noticed because in the midst of her struggle with Timothy, she said, "Wow, you're always pushing out lessons with your son, aren't you?"

I was interacting with Giaci by asking questions about the colour of objects we saw, asking him to point to things, and any other teachable moment that came up was never overlooked.

"This is how I was trained as a teacher. Learning happens at all times, so I try as best I can whenever possible to do that," I responded. I knew that constant learning was fundamental, and we had an entire behavioural team working with him after Shipu left. I had learned from being a teacher and from watching his team of therapists.

After a few minutes of waiting, Dr. Krone entered the room. She greeted us with a matronly stance, and her voice was calming.

"Hello, everyone," she said, greeting Janice, Hope and me. She glanced around the room and paid extra attention to Giaci and Timothy. Her tone even soothed Timothy for a moment.

After brief introductions, she got right down to business. "I've looked over your sons' bloodwork with my colleagues and our pediatrics team. Together, we've created a plan." She passed us each our individual portfolios. "Research has shown that by using basic blood chemistry blended with lipid bench science and a targeted nutritional intervention, we should see improvements in both your sons' development."

I was trying to take it all in, but Timothy started to fuss again. Hope took him for a walk so that Janice could give her undivided attention to Dr. Krone.

Once the two were gone, Dr. Krone continued. "This program involves biomedical interventions and targeted nutritional interventions, which means there will be a level of commitment and focus on your part?" She finished her sentence as if it was a question. Janice and I looked at each other; neither of us was a stranger to doing whatever it took. We both nodded.

After a routine exam of our boys, we were given a package of paperwork, liquids, and supplements, as well as forms for when we depleted these supplies. The costs were not mentioned, but I assumed it was in all the paperwork. Neither Janice nor I brought it up; we were just focusing on the possibilities of helping our sons. We did not want to focus on the cost of it all in that moment. For me, when it came to Giaci's health and well-being, everything else fell to the sidelines.

On the flight home I began reading all the papers, overwhelmed by how much this could change our lives—and then I spotted the cost, which stung my eyes as I read on.

THIRTY

A Mother's Wishful Thinking

Giaci's new diet brought a brisk shift to our lives. We had to start him on a gluten- and casein-free diet and had to make sure he took the necessary supplements and electrolytes. I didn't want to miss a thing, so I wrote it all down in a notebook, recording everything he ingested, including the amount I gave him, the time it was given, and any observations I made about his physical and behavioural reactions to the food.

Even more difficult, there weren't many products available that would fit his new restrictive diet. I asked a local baker if he would make Giaci gluten- and casein-free bread and muffins. This wasn't the only difference in Giaci's diet; all of his meals were different from the rest of the family's, which was a challenge to say the least.

He would often launch himself at our plates, trying to grab the food the rest of us were eating. Giaci was masterful at sneaking food right from under our noses. The minute I took my eyes off him, he would take the opportunity to devour whatever was in reach. His speed and precision were remarkable.

Eventually Lauren was forced to eat her crackers in the closet, and Carolina and Maria became the tattletale police. If Giaci was attempting to take food that he wasn't supposed to eat, one of them would sound the alarm.

"Mommy! Giaci is climbing up onto the counter. He's trying to eat the bread from inside the cupboard!" they wailed, pointing at him. I couldn't blame them; they were doing all they could to be my watchful eyes.

If I had to run to the bathroom, Giaci knew it was his chance to make a break for the cookies on the top shelf of the pantry. That's when the tag team would spring into action. Carolina was usually the first to notice that her brother was going for the forbidden gluten-rich food. Maria was the runner who, once her sister tipped her off, would take the virtual baton and rush over to notify me of the situation. Poor Giaci didn't stand a chance with all the police cadets in our house.

Going to visit anyone became extremely difficult because of all the gluten and casein temptations awaiting in Italian households. Any event we attended had an abundance of these foods that we were adamantly trying to stay away from. For Italians, forbidding family members from sharing their food with Giaci could be viewed as offensive.

The two nonnas tried making rice pasta, but it wasn't the satisfying and delicious Italian food they were accustomed to serving. The one time my mom made it, she expressed disgust; it didn't taste as good or look as appealing.

Wearing an apron that depicted the island of Sicily, my mom usually started the cooking process early in the morning, first sauteing the onions and garlic. Then she added the jarred tomatoes and some fresh herbs from the garden and allowed it to simmer on low most of the day. The aroma filled the house, and as soon as Giaci arrived, his eyes opened wide. He knew Nonna was making either lasagna or pasta with her homemade sauce.

"Let him have some. Just one bowl." She felt that I was being a hard-ass about it and that I should be more lenient, but I had to be strict to see the full effects of this program. It didn't matter how much I explained the reason for this diet; she was under the impression that I was depriving my son.

"I'm not doing this to hurt him, Ma! This is to help him." I tried to explain the link between food and the brain, but in her eyes, I was tormenting both her and Giaci. Since the effects of this special diet weren't visible immediately—or at all—it seemed useless to the nonnas.

This particular day, we were having penne. It was his most desired food, a pasta much celebrated in Italian cuisine.

It was hard to convince Giaci that the other food was just as delicious as his nonna's, especially since his grandparents didn't quite understand what we were trying to do.

"Just a little, *nan dichia*. I'll give him just a little bit." My mom split his plate between the two versions, the rice pasta and the regular pasta. It was clear to Giaci which was which, and he barely touched the rice pasta.

At least my mom was gentler in her approach; Nonna Carolina was more aggressive in filling his bowl to the top.

"*Te, fallo mangiare*, let him eat," she said. She fixed her eyes on Giaci, watching him indulge, and then shifted them to me, as if I hadn't fed him in weeks.

"Eh, see? He lovey *mia* pasta!" Her words were like a slap. For her, it was satisfying to see how Giaci loved and devoured her pasta. Her food was desired, which was her love language.

I tried to explain our objectives to the best of my ability, but I never seemed to get through to them. Visits became that much more tiring. We didn't want to offend, but we also had to stay true to our mission. As a result, we chose to visit family members less and less often, which was taken out of context as being disrespectful. When we did visit, it was after having eaten at home. We resorted to short, late visits to find a middle ground. We weren't trying to be insulting; we just wanted to improve our son's digestion and leaky gut syndrome. We continued to stay the course as best we could and put the displeased reactions on the shelf for another day.

We had to enforce the dietary restrictions, and we also had a specific nutritional regimen to follow. At first, the daily round of nutritional supplements and electrolytes was difficult to administer as Giaci gave us a hard time. I had to enforce the "first this, then that" method. This worked for us before with fruits and vegetables, so we applied this technique to his new diet and supplements.

In time, he accepted the regimen of taking the supplements one at a time without any fuss. It was a slow process of encouragement and verbal praise, but worth it. I would put the supplements on a napkin with a glass of water beside it, and Giaci knew he had to put them in his mouth and wash them down with the water, just like adults did.

My trust in this process was buoyed when, after weeks of analyzing and controlling Giaci's nutritional intake, I witnessed a slight change in his disposition. It was faint, but I was convinced that it happened, and it was mind-boggling. Giaci had always seemed to live a foggy existence; his eye contact was minimal, and his responses to my interactions were limited and forced. Then, one day, I noticed a shift.

He was playing on the swing set in our fenced backyard, enjoying the back-and-forth motion and the wind blowing against his face. His sisters were running around him, playing a game of tag. Lauren was the tallest but not the fastest, so Maria and Carolina would often tag her without much trouble. I watched the natural interaction of the girls playing while keeping a close eye on Giaci. I would call to him from the deck, but he didn't respond with words or actions. He liked to keep to himself while playing in his own world. Still, day after day I called out to him, to maintain consistency.

"Buddy! You look like you're having fun! Hi, Giaci!" I called.

This time, he looked directly at me.

Once I realized that I had gotten his attention, I started jumping up and down on the deck. "Giaci! You hear me? Hi, Giaci!" I waved dramatically.

Then I heard his beautiful response.

"Hi, Mommy!" he said from his spot on the swing before jumping off and running around the backyard like he was racing Usain Bolt doing laps on a track.

I was thrilled by his interaction. It was a marginal step in the right direction.

"Giaci, where are you?" I asked, trying to test his response time.

"Here I am," he answered after a few moments.

Every day after that, I noticed him using a little more language. He was laying eyes *on* me rather than looking *through* me. When he saw my expressive and overjoyed expression, his face radiated. He wanted to please me.

A rush of excitement came over me. My motivation ignited like never before; all I could think of was doing everything I could to push things forward to reveal his true personality. I had been skeptical of this outcome, but now it felt possible. We were moving forward on intensive behavioural intervention with a new team of therapists, and his gluten-and casein-free diet and a very strict regimen of nutritional supplements seemed to be working.

Every week, Janice and I talked on the phone, discussing our sons' progress.

"I see changes in Timothy," she said. "He is more alert, and his digestive problems, like bloating, diarrhea, and gas, are all better than before. I can't believe it." I could hear the hope and enthusiasm in her voice.

"Giaci is showing improvements too. His eye contact has improved, and I'm noticing more language. He is interacting with his sisters more," I said.

It was satisfying and even exhilarating to have someone else to share this experience with. For so long I had felt alone, unable to connect or share these sorts of experiences with anyone other than John. With Janice, I could share emotions, aspirations and stories. We were like giddy teenagers, chatting away on the phone and giving each other updates. We were bonding and felt like we were off on our own adventure.

THIRTY-ONE

A Horrific Night

On most days, our household was a messy flurry of activity. Today, the kids provided an energetic and noisy backdrop while I interviewed new behaviour therapists for Giaci after school. Due to the government-imposed age restriction on their intensive behaviour intervention therapy services, we were back to paying privately and introducing strangers into the house. John trusted me to conduct the interviews while he continued to go from job site to job site. I was used to taking the reins on all things Giaci-related.

The only therapist I'd interviewed who stood out was Agapi. A friend had said that she was "a hard worker and patient." These were traits I ranked high on my list of wants in an instructor-therapist.

After calling Agapi and offering her the job, it was time to get the kids ready for dinner. Darkness came early, so even though it was dinnertime, it felt much later.

Giaci still turned up his nose at the gluten-free pasta, even when it was drizzled with homemade tomato sauce, but he did eat gluten-free crackers. We hadn't been sticking to the entire intense diet for about three months, as it became too complicated for the whole family, but there were parts that stuck. He liked the crackers and rice and almond milk.

Giaci now sat at the table and ate with ease by himself. Looking at his lipstick of tomato sauce and the wide smile on his face, I seized the opportunity to run downstairs to the basement to finish laundry, as I had many times before. On my way down the stairs, I got a call from

John, letting me know he had to run to the hardware store and that he wouldn't be long. This was the norm; we were all busy doing something.

I didn't want to stay downstairs for long, so as soon as I finished folding the laundry, I threw in another load and dashed past Lauren, who was in the basement on the couch reading a book. I ran upstairs and passed the twins, who were playing with their Beanie Baby dolls.

When I walked into the kitchen to check on Giaci, I found a half-eaten bowl of pasta and an empty chair. This was odd because he would always finish his bowl of pasta and ask for more.

"Giaci?" I called out, even though I knew he didn't always react or respond to being called. I searched the house, hurdling over toys and bins, thinking he had gone into another room, but I didn't find him.

Intense heat flickered up my body. My worst fear was coming true.

"Giaci! Giaci, answer me!" I barreled through rooms crying and screeching his name without any response.

Oh my God, where is he? My stomach churned.

I panted as my heart pulsed through my skin. He was chronologically six years old but cognitively functioned at less than half his age. He couldn't fend for himself. He wouldn't even be able to communicate with anyone. The realization pinched the hairs on the back of my neck, and my legs collapsed underneath me. Cement blocks bolted me down, but they couldn't hold in the scream that burst throughout the house.

"What's wrong, Mommy?" Suddenly Lauren was beside me, one small hand on my thigh while the other still held her book.

I barely heard her question. "Lauren, stay here with the twins. Mommy has to go outside to find Giaci."

Her face fell. She knew this was serious.

Though the thought of leaving my three little girls alone was petrifying, I had no choice. I had to search for my son.

The girls are safe. The girls are safe. I gasped for air as I opened the front door and stepped out onto the porch. I didn't see any neighbours, though. It was like a ghost town; everyone was sitting inside peacefully for their evening meal while I howled with the wind outside. I could hear the crunch of the sleet under the rubber of my shoes. The smell of the pine trees around me made the blackness even darker.

I began to run through the neighbourhood. *He has to be close. I wasn't gone that long.* The words blazing through my head were the only things keeping me grounded. I couldn't maintain my composure. I probably looked frantic to the neighbours, sprinting from the front yard to the back and all around the block.

There was no sign of him, no glimpse of him anywhere. Then I thought, *Maybe John took him to the hardware store with him. Maybe I didn't hear him because of the loud sounds from the washing machine and dryer.* Thinking back, I realized that I hadn't heard the door alarm that would beep every time we opened and closed a door.

I had forgotten my cellphone, so I ran back home to call John. I noticed that Giaci's shoes were gone from the foyer. At one time, this would have indicated that either John or I had dressed him, but we'd recently taught him to put on his own Velcro shoes, so he may still have gone out on his own.

I choked on failing hope. Out of breath, I called John's cell.

"John, do you have Giaci?" There was a brief silence.

"No, where is he?" For once, John's voice rose in worry.

As soon as he said those words, I fell back, hitting the wall, and screamed, "I'm calling 911." As I dialed, the most horrific thoughts overwhelmed me. Giaci running through the dark streets. Giaci getting hurt. The unimaginable.

When the 911 operator answered, I gasped for air and immediately began rambling. "My son is missing. He has autism and is a runner and has limited language and *please* help me find him! *Please!*" I was bawling by the end of this rant. There was a painful, piercing pinch in the middle of my throat.

The 911 operator asked me several questions:

"How old is your son, and what was he wearing?"

I shook my head from left to right, as if to help my brain focus on his appearance. I steadied my breath and tried to calm my rising panic to give her a description.

"He's six years old and has a blue Adidas T-shirt and…grey Tommy Hilfiger sweatpants."

"What colour hair and eyes?" she asked.

"He has…green eyes and short, light-brown hair. Oh my God," I said, stomping my feet impatiently. "Please, we have to find him! Please! I'll answer your questions, but can you please send people now?" I begged.

"I understand, ma'am, but I need you to answer my questions so we can have a better chance of finding him," the responder calmly reassured me. She paused and I could hear click-clacking on her keyboard as quickly as my feet were tapping.

Within minutes, she told me that a boy had been found matching Giaci's description. "Ma'am, I believe we have your son."

I put my hand over my mouth to stifle a scream. I struggled to hold my head straight.

"Mrs. Miceli, your son was found in the middle of a busy street, three blocks from your home. An elderly couple was walking by and noticed him. They took him back to their home and called the authorities." Her voice hesitated periodically as she regurgitated the information in front of her. "After the elderly couple called the police, arrangements were made to have your son put into foster care." Horror was replaced with anger as I thought about my baby boy being taken into custody.

I collapsed onto the carpeted steps by the front door, still pressing the phone to my ear with my trembling hand. I stifled a gut-wrenching shriek.

As if she could hear me fall, the 911 operator said, "Sorry, ma'am. This is standard protocol."

Even though it seemed like forever since Giaci had disappeared from the house, it couldn't have been longer than thirty minutes. Why were they already planning for foster care?

"Where is he? I'll go get him. I'll be there in five minutes."

Just as the dispatcher informed me that the police would escort Giaci home, John burst through the door. His eyes were bulging out of his head, and he was panting with pulsing adrenalin.

"Please hurry!" I screamed at the phone before darting toward John.

He opened his arms and squeezed me as we both wept in a firm embrace. We were stunned and emotionally drained. The girls watched us from the living room, crying from our shared tumultuous experience. If I could have split myself between John and my children, I would have embraced the girls as well.

After sharing an emotional release with John, I opened the front door and we stood on our small square cement porch, anticipating our son's return, despite the bitter Canadian winter. From the porch, we could see our girls peering anxiously out through the front window.

John couldn't speak. There were no words. The colour had drained from his face; he was clearly stunned by the mass confusion of our son's disappearance. For once, six-foot-tall John looked defeated and small, no matter how much he tried to be brave for us all.

Finally, I could see flickering lights brightening our street. Soon after, the police cruiser parked curbside in front of our house. The previously shadowy neighbours came to their windows to peer out, likely wondering what was happening over at the Micelis' house.

When the police car stopped and the officers climbed out, I darted out onto the stiff grass to grab Giaci. As John and I approached the police car, the policeman raised his palm.

"You need to step back," he said in a firm, deep voice, motioning again with his hand.

My entire body trembled from withdrawal. I just needed to hug my baby.

"Is this your son?" the officer asked.

"Yes, that's my son, yes!" I answered.

He kept his watchful eyes on me and without emotion said, "I'll open the door."

Giaci was in the back seat of the police car, his little arms wrapped around a brown teddy bear. He was smiling, amused and carefree as he often was. I let out my first full smile when I saw his bright face. A cold sweat still poured down my forehead, and every instinct in me roared to go to him. I was unable to contain my nurturing and protective instinct, and when I started to move closer, ready to snatch my child from the police car, John wrapped his strong arms around me.

"He's okay. Look, he's coming," he whispered in my ear. To the officers, it would have looked like an embrace and not a desperate restraint.

"Giaci, what did you do? Why did you leave Mommy?" I called out, but he didn't answer. Instead, he continued smiling and slowly ambled over me, oblivious to the magnitude of my distress. Giaci had had the time of his life on this adventure, and to top it off, the policemen had rewarded him with a prize: a teddy bear. They had no idea what they'd done. Giaci giggled and glowed, satisfied with the night's events.

Once he was in front of me, I lunged down to hug him. "Mommy loves you so much. Oh, you scared me!" I looked up from our sweet embrace and saw the judging eyes of the officers.

Within seconds, I felt John securely wrap his arms around us both.

One of the officers cleared his throat. "We're going to have to come in and ask you some questions."

They stiffly followed us into our home. We didn't make it halfway into the foyer before they began their interrogation.

"We need to understand what happened here this evening," the lead officer said, frowning at us.

I felt like the worst mother on earth. How could I have let this happen? How?

John zeroed in on my drained expression and took the lead.

"Officers, my wife was busy tending to our three daughters, and I had gone to the hardware store. My son has autism, and he left our house without anyone noticing."

I continued to whimper softly, holding Giaci at my side.

"Has this ever happened before?" the officer asked, jotting notes down in his little booklet.

"No, never," John said.

Their exchange continued for about twenty long minutes. Obliterated, I went to the couch and sat motionless surrounded by my four children. Lauren pulled at her hair while the twins stood like soldiers, unwilling to leave my side.

Once the policemen were satisfied with John's answers, they said, "Okay, we will write up our report. Goodbye." And then they went on their way. Before closing the door, John thanked them for helping us recover our son. Almost immediately, John deadbolted the door behind them and leaned on it for a moment, trying to catch his breath.

The twins couldn't help but stare as the men left; their eyes were big and bothered as they followed the officers through the window until they got back into their vehicle. Even at a young age, they understood the seriousness of the officers' presence and that something was wrong. Lauren focused her attention on her brother and sat beside him, clenching his hand tightly. She was his unyielding protector.

I still couldn't believe what had happened. We were tasered by the events yet realized that it could have been far, far worse. Giaci could have been killed. We were thankful he was alive and back in our home, but my mind couldn't rest.

"He could have died! He was found in the middle of a busy street! John! He could have died!" My body found the energy for another moment of hysteria. It set off a chain reaction in the girls, and we all sobbed together.

John quickly regained his composure and helped us with ours.

"Rita, he didn't die. He's here, we have him back, and we aren't going to let this happen again."

He came over to rub my back, but all my anger was still coming out full force. I ran far from John and the girls to let it out. The back wall of the kitchen was my victim as I punched and kicked at it. I needed the physical contact to feel like I was still alive. Everything else was so numb, and with each punch I felt more in control. When my hands were bruised, I ran to my room, sobbing.

From my room, even over my crying, I could hear John tucking the kids into bed. I heard him go into the garage to grab tools. I couldn't settle myself down, so I got up to see what he was doing. With his electric drill, he was screwing in a latch onto the front door, high enough so that the kids couldn't reach it. He also added a lock to the back door, securing our home in the front and back. I stood frozen, only able to move my hands to wipe the tears that dripped off my face. I still felt numb, as if nothing that was happening was real.

Once John had finished with his drill, he shut all the lights off and walked me back to bed. He held me tight all night long as if it would ease the pain, but it didn't. Every time I came close to falling asleep, I startled awake, wondering if Giaci had run off again. I wanted to check on him, but John convinced me not to wake him.

"He can't get out. That lock will keep him—and us—safe," he cooed before falling back to sleep.

John was reassured, but I wasn't. Replaying Giaci's buoyancy in the back of the police cruiser, I knew this wouldn't be the last time he would attempt to run away. It had been a positive experience for him, and the reward for this behaviour would entice him to do it again. I feared reliving this nightmarish evening.

I lay awake the entire night, revisited by negative thoughts I'd believed I'd vanquished. Depression swept over me, pressing me down, reminding me that it was always a breath away. No matter how far I'd come, it was just around the corner, waiting to strike, watching for an inevitable moment of weakness.

Terror had broken me. I would never be the same.

THIRTY-TWO

"What Will Others Think" Syndrome

After a night spent with negative thoughts, I was in no shape to go to work the next day. I laid in bed dreading the call I'd have to make to the principal, the one where I'd have to relive the traumatic experience all over again.

Giaci attended the school where I worked, and I understood that the Children's Aid Society (CAS) would be contacting the school. As a teacher, I knew that it was standard protocol for CAS to follow up with the child's school after receiving a police report. But being the parent on the other end of that notification was mortifying. How could anyone question our motives when it came to Giaci? How could anyone think we would harm our own son?

The school would know everything even before I made the call. All my co-workers would know that Giaci had run away from home. Shame engulfed me and pulled me back under the covers for a moment. I forced a breath in, pulling the duvet off, which was wet with my tears. I welcomed the stifled air.

The "What Will Others Think" syndrome reared up within me again, but this time I couldn't run from it. Everyone would know what had happened. I couldn't pretend or wish otherwise. I picked up the phone to call the principal.

"Hello, Catia. I won't be in today," I said.

"You okay? What's wrong, Rita?" she replied.

"I'm still trying to wrap my head around what happened to us last night," I told her, then filled her in on what had happened. In between my moments of silence, I tried to compose myself. I knew she would get the police report today, so I wanted her to hear it from me first. She was more sympathetic than I'd been with myself.

"I'm so sorry you had to go through this, Rita," Catia said. Her tender words cushioned me as she added, "I'm so relieved to hear that he's home safe with you. Take the day and let me know if there's anything we can do for you." Her understanding brought me some peace. She made me feel like it could have happened to anyone.

As I hung up with Catia, John, the girls and Giaci began trickling down the hallway, ready to start their day. They were all cheery faces and sleepy eyes; none of them looked like I did. There was no hint of crying, no echo of the screams of the night before, just their usual waking faces and morning greetings, followed by our mundane routines and rituals.

I instinctively went into mommy autopilot, buttering toast, helping the kids get washed and dressed for the day. John had important meetings scheduled throughout his workday, and he was going to cancel his afternoon to spend time at home with us. I needed him to. Dressed in his navy-blue suit, he calmly approached me and once again wrapped his strong arms around my body. This morning's hug lasted longer than usual. It lingered with knowing.

"We will get through this, Rita, one step at a time. We will, for Giaci and for our family." His bravery resonated even through his whisper. He had put the events of the previous night behind him and made the conscious decision to move forward.

After he left for the office, I deadbolted the door and fastened the extra latch for greater protection. None of us were going to school or daycare this day. I went downstairs with the kids and put a movie on for them. Plopping myself on the couch behind them, I tried to relax my sore, aching body. I had physical symptoms from the emotional trauma. Muscle tension, joint pain, a headache, and chest pain. I couldn't fully relax. Paranoia poked me every minute; Giaci had to be in view and arms' reach. I knew that with the TV on, he wouldn't run off, but I couldn't rationalize my way out of this panic spiral.

When I did finally doze off, flashes of busy streets with cars zooming past Giaci assaulted my psyche. I jolted awake and didn't see him, which immediately set my heart racing. I let out a yelp, alerting the girls, who were still enjoying their special TV time. Lauren, who knew I was still shaken from the night before, pointed to the far end of the room, where Giaci was running from wall to wall. I moved to break his course, and he ran right into me, propelling us into a monster hug. For as long as he let me, I held him, trying not to sob. John was right. Giaci was here, and he was safe. I couldn't break again…not like before. Staring into Giaci's captivating grass-coloured eyes, I found my motivation. I found strength in my love for him. He was always motivating me to do more.

I thought about our current situation and how recently we had been bouncing back and forth between therapists for Giaci. We offered part-time hours, so our workers were students. After Agapi finished her university education, she found work elsewhere as a speech therapist and left our employment. We hired Ashley, another student, and paid a clinical psychologist, Dr. Barrera, to train her.

Six months later, when Ashley finished her schooling and began working full-time as a nurse, we were left having to hire another new person to work with Giaci.

Before leaving us, Ashley mentioned that her younger sister and her friend would be interested. After meeting Megan and Kelly, I made the arrangements to have them trained in behavioural intervention by our clinical psychologist, Dr. Barrera, as well. Soon after, Jessica was another addition to Giaci's team.

They knew how to record the necessary data and implement the task-analysis system we were using. Each step of a given task that was being taught was implemented exactly the same way so there was no confusion for Giaci.

With each new therapist, Giaci took time to adjust to a new presence, as did the rest of our family—and there was the financial strain we incurred. Giaci's progress was slow and steady, which is what mattered most. He was saying more words and interacting more frequently.

Janice and I didn't speak as regularly. Six months had passed since the last time I called her; she had brushed me off because she was busy at work and had her hands full with Timothy. We were both juggling our days as best we could, but I did miss our chats.

* * *

I often thought of my father's words, telling me how important education was.

After putting the kids to bed at night, I would scour the internet searching for something else to learn about autism. I came across a few educational forums. The one that caught my attention was a three-day symposium on autism in Toronto at the Geneva Centre for Autism. This symposium was bringing in experts from all over the world to speak. I signed up on the spot and then worked out the details with John.

The symposium was three weeks away. The thought of being away for several days was unsettling, but as soon as I told John about the workshops, he rearranged his schedule to take over my child-rearing duties, no justification or explanation needed. Whatever I told him I wanted to do for our children, he supported beyond measure, especially for Giaci.

The morning I left for Toronto was brisk, and the weathered train station was packed. I had my luggage, complete with books to read on the train and paper and pens to take notes. I was ready to be fully enlightened. It was a four-hour train ride, which gave me the opportunity to finish reading a family's inspirational story about living with autism.

The book was *Let Me Hear Your Voice* by Catherine Maurice, a mother who had two children diagnosed with autism. The story details the agony and heartbreak she and her husband experienced as they struggled to help their children "recover" from autism.

This book inspired me as I connected with her story; I, too, wanted my son to recover from autism.

* * *

When I arrived in Toronto, I took a taxi to the hotel, which was right next to the venue for the symposium. I dropped off my suitcase before registering for the individual sessions with the speakers I wanted to hear. There were so many important sessions being offered, it was difficult to decide which sessions to join. I wanted to absorb as much information as I could within those three days.

Temple Grandin was one of the presenters; she was the most famous individual on the autism spectrum who had documented the insights she'd gained from her own personal experience with the condition. I made sure to get to the conference room for her talk early because I wanted to secure a preferred seat.

As I sat waiting for Temple to start, I glanced around, watching hundreds of people assemble into the spacious room. I wondered if they were all parents like me, living a similar life with autism. After spending so much time isolated, it was hard to fathom that there were hundreds like our family.

Soon an announcer introduced Temple, and then she strolled onto the stage. She looked exactly like her photo in her book.

Prior to going to Toronto, I had read *Thinking in Pictures*. I'd even brought it with me, hoping to have her sign it. Temple stood about nine feet away from me, dressed in jeans, leather cowboy boots, a checkered cowboy shirt, and a skinny scarf-like bow tied around her neck. Her shirt was tucked into her pants so that her brown leather belt could be seen.

She appeared comfortable and natural, with no makeup.

When she began speaking, I was impressed with how she was able to express herself and tell her story. Her Midwestern accent would rise and lower at unexpected times, and she would accentuate certain words in ways I had never heard before. She spoke with her hands a lot, just like an Italian, and I grinned at the similarity. She had this way of making everyone in the room feel comfortable.

I was captivated by her storytelling. She explained her ability to think in specific, photographic images. She had a sharp visual acuity, seeing videos play in her imagination, and she excelled at visual spatial skills. She viewed the world differently than most, yet her ability bridged our world and hers, allowing us a glimpse into a different sort of mind.

"The worst thing you can do is nothing," she said, referring to teaching children with autism. That was my philosophy as well. As I listened to her, I thought of my son. Did Giaci see the world like Temple? Giaci couldn't communicate nearly as well as she did. She blatantly stated that she had not "recovered" from autism but had learned, through huge effort, to adapt to the social norms of the people around her.

"If I could snap my fingers and be non-autistic, I would not. Autism is part of what I am, of who I am," she said, which resonated with me.

Even though she had lived through many difficulties, her autism had given her so many incredible abilities. Since Giaci's initial diagnosis, all I'd wanted was to rid him of his autism. Maybe I'd been missing something.

Temple explained how her mother had "stretched her," exposing her to many different things, and how that had affected her learning in her life. We were constantly stretching Giaci with new foods. There were always new experiences for him. We focused on more learning…endless learning, it seemed.

"Eye contact is still difficult for me in noisy rooms because it interferes with hearing," Temple said. "It's like my brain's wiring lets only one sense function over the others, but sometimes not at the same time. In noisy rooms I have to concentrate on hearing." She had finally put into words something I'd noticed with Giaci.

After an incredible hour of listening to her speak about her successful life and passion for livestock-handling facilities and animal behaviour, I wanted to meet her. Temple announced that if anyone wanted her autograph, she would be signing books after her presentation. When she was finished, I approached the line that quickly formed to have my copy autographed.

When it was my turn, I stepped toward her small table, watching Temple manoeuvre a black Sharpie pen in her hand. I handed her my book and expressed my admiration for her success and how she embraced her abilities.

She turned to me and asked, "Should I make it out to Rita?" as if we already knew each other.

Baffled, I looked down at my name tag. I was wearing a black fleece jacket, unzipped, which covered part of my blue Nike T-shirt. My name tag was on the right side of my T-shirt, still covered by my jacket. With a small gasp of confusion, I said, "Yes, please," and watched her autograph my book. As I stood watching and waiting for her to finish signing my book, I replayed the scene in my head, trying to figure out how she knew my name. It was as if she had performed an incredible magic trick.

When she had finished signing my copy of her book, I thanked her and walked away, star-struck and dumbfounded. The only conclusion I could come up with was that when I was in line, I had turned for a brief moment—a split second, really—to peer behind me to see the length of the line. With that quick movement, my jacket must have moved, exposing my name tag. Temple, having a heightened visual ability, must have seen my name tag while she was still talking to the lady in front of me.

I turned once more to take a final peek at her, my eyes wide. I was blown away that she had applied her incredible visual abilities to me. I smiled, noticing her attentive eyes studying me as I moved farther away.

At the symposium, there was an Autism Ontario booth. I approached the person at the booth, hoping to gain more insights. This woman was a volunteer. She informed me about a meeting organized by Autism Ontario. This meeting would have two guest speakers, both provincial government officials. She recommended I go because it was going to be about the government autism services. It was going to take place at another hotel, so I had to jump into a taxi to get there. It was scheduled to take place in two hours, so I grabbed a quick bite and flagged down a taxi.

Once the taxi driver entered the hotel parking lot, he noticed a mob of people with signs.

"Wow, what's going on here?" he asked, not knowing where to drop me off.

I assumed that it had to do with the meeting I was attending. The two government officials who were speaking made and implemented decisions on policies regarding autism services.

I asked the driver to let me out at the curb, paid him, and hopped out. As he drove off, I turned toward the crowd, wondering if they would allow me entry. Taking a deep breath, I proceeded with caution. I made my way through the crowd of people, who were chanting and holding up signs.

Age is but a number!
My child is worth it!
Invest now so it's less later!
ABA best outcome!

There were many more I couldn't see. Their protesting resonated powerfully with me, as I lived in a similar situation with the age cutoff. A few signs had pictures of the protestors' own children displayed on them, which added impact. I gave a thumbs-up to one mom as I squeezed past her. Luckily, I was able to get to the door without anyone blocking my path, but the security guard wanted to see my registration forms. This was a special meeting for members of Autism Ontario who had previously registered. There was a limit to the number of people allowed to attend, and I was fortunate to have registered early enough to be one of them.

After verifying my legitimacy, the guard directed me where to go. The multicoloured carpeted hallway led me to the assigned meeting room. A woman sat on a stackable chair by a table, asking that everyone sign in before entering.

"Hello and welcome," she said, like I was going to see a Broadway play. "Please sign and print your name right here and indicate if you are a parent or a professional." She gestured to where to sign and give my information.

I signed the form and noticed that many others had also signed in as parents. Once again, I wasn't alone in my quest to advocate for my child. In fact, from what I saw, it was mainly parents in attendance. Parents from all over the province of Ontario wanted to hear from these two politicians, the Minister of Education and the Minister of Community and Youth Services. This meeting was to discuss the expansion of services for children with autism, specifically the age-six cut-off for intervention therapy.

Even though we lived in a country with universal health care, these behavioural services were not considered "medical," so they were not covered. It was only after a great deal of pressure from parents that the government implemented their behavioural intervention services for children ages five to six—services which I had already fought to extend as part of the class-action lawsuit.

The meeting was late to begin, and the chatter among the crowd became more heated as we waited. As I turned to look at the doorway, I saw the ministers enter, strutting along in their professional business suits. The crowd scoffed at them. Everyone around me was tense and angry. These politicians had the power to impact lives, and I too was infuriated by how they handled it. I didn't know them, and they didn't know me, yet they had the power to affect the trajectory of not only my son's life but also my entire family's life. They had the ability to give my son the services he needed. And they wouldn't.

The ministers sat on a riser with a table in front of them. They leaned forward in their chairs, placing their elbows on the table. I was perhaps ten feet away, sitting in the sea of chairs facing them.

The provincial president of Autism Ontario introduced the ministers to the rowdy crowd.

"Ladies and gentlemen, we are fortunate to have with us today two provincial ministers, the Minister of Education and the Minister of Community and Youth Services. There will be a question period at the end of this meeting, so please hold your comments and questions until then. I ask for your undivided attention! Please give them a warm welcome," she boomed, which was followed only by a subdued clap.

Then the crowd went silent.

Everyone focused on the information the government officials shared. The minister with russet-coloured hair took the lead. She spoke in a true charismatic tone, stating what her government had already done and what they were going to do. I tried to understand her political rhetoric, but all I could focus on was what I wanted and needed for my son. My doubts overpowered my belief in her. When would she address the fact that Giaci had been on a waitlist for almost two years and now, because of his age, was being cut off from services? We had to privately pay our behavioural team of therapists to continue. These costs were difficult to maintain, and no family should have to go through what we were facing. Most families couldn't even begin to pay for these treatments.

When the minister proudly informed us that their two ministries were now working together to provide more services for children with autism, I inwardly groaned. I wanted to stand up and shut her down. She needed to understand how tired we all were of the "all talk and no action" reality! My body heat rose along with my blood pressure, and with a flushed face I cringed at their hollow words.

Then the blonde minister jumped in, telling the crowd that IBI would be provided to children up to the age of six. With a resounding voice, she said into the microphone:

"The school system will begin receiving training on behavioural strategies. Once the child has finished IBI services at age six, he or she will enter the education system and receive continued behavioural teachings there. This way, what was started at home will continue seamlessly in the schools."

As an educator, I knew that the school system did not provide ABA or IBI. Educators in the school system didn't have training in this type of intervention, which was imperative. The education system was not ready to address my son's needs, and I couldn't have Giaci losing the one and only kind of therapy that showed promise.

After the two ministers finished speaking, they opened the floor for questions. The audience got rowdier as people hurried to assemble in a line behind the microphone. I was determined to speak my truth. I had much to say, and I wanted them to hear it. I was the voice for my son, and I needed to advocate for him. I sprang out of my seat and stood, hands on my hips, in my spot in the long line of mothers and fathers. We were limited to one question each, but most of us had the same questions.

"My son has been on the waitlist to receive IBI services for two years. When will the age restriction be lifted?" the first mother asked. She stood strong in her convictions and wore a T-shirt with her child's face on it. With her feet planted, she sent the strong message that she was ready for some kind of change.

Emotions were at an all-time high in the room. Parents were scoffing. The tension was visible. Punch by punch, blow by blow, the politicians were hit with questions and disappointment. As seasoned politicians, the two women answered every question with reassurance, offering support and understanding. They were effective communicators and did not beat around the bush. They were direct in their messaging, using diverse pitches and intensities in their voices.

I waited through every question, refining my agitated thoughts into a coherent question. *I'm going to have my say*, I thought as the line slowly advanced. Inch by inch, I felt closer to saying my piece. My voice would be heard. I was next.

Then a representative from Autism Ontario announced that our time had ended. The meeting was over. She added placatingly:

"If anyone has any further questions, please forward them to me and I'll follow up with a response from the ministers as quickly as I can." Her voice echoed from the speakers around the room.

I grew hot and developed tunnel vision. I hadn't been given a chance to ask my question! The two ministers hadn't seen me. I wanted to be noticed and remembered. *This discussion isn't over*, I thought.

Unwilling to accept being muted, I watched as the two politicians were escorted out by their entourage and security. I grabbed my heavy bag. I was on a mission to plead my son's case. I found myself following them out of the conference room. The education minister and her people dashed out the side door to a van that was waiting for them. As the possibility of talking to her ended abruptly, I immediately turned in the other direction and focused on the Minister of Community and Youth Services. She was walking toward the restroom, so I followed. I had this one opportunity before she would disappear as well. There was only one thing to do.

I approached the security guard stationed outside the bathroom door and said, "Hello! I'm so sorry, but I really have to go to the bathroom," with the most sincere and genuine voice I could.

The oversized man turned and studied me, questioning my true intent.

I reiterated, "I really have to go. I promise I won't be long." I gave my best performance yet, with sweetness all over my face.

I must have seemed harmless because he nodded and let me pass. He could never have known that there was a mama wolf under that sheepskin. As I opened the door and entered the bathroom, I didn't see anyone at first, but then I noticed that one stall door was closed. I turned in the other direction and saw my reflection in the mirror. There was a new expression on my face. It was the likeness of a mother who was ready to cause a ruckus for her family when she needed to.

I washed my hands as I waited for the minister to finish in the stall. Doubt began to wash over me. What was I doing following this woman into the bathroom? She was going to have me arrested. As I pondered my reckless actions driven by sheer emotion, I heard the squeak of the stall door opening.

She reappeared.

She noticed me there.

Our eyes made contact, and she squeezed her upper and lower lips together, giving me a brief nod, acknowledging my presence. As I grabbed a paper towel to dry my hands, I turned and glanced at her. I pretended to be surprised, dramatically lifting my facial features and pulling out my best version of Actress Rita.

"Oh! Hello, Minister! I know this is an awkward place to speak, but if I could just take a moment of your time, please?" I said in the most straightforward and honest way I could.

She approached the sink to wash her hands and hesitantly said, "Yes, of course."

That was my green light. But instead of releasing my inner mama wolf, I found myself not wanting to blow the whole house down. I wanted her to see the genuine anguish and humanity in my face. I didn't want my son to be a number on her list. I wanted her to know our story and be affected by the real struggles we faced because of her decisions.

"Thank you for listening, Minister. My son has autism, and he was cut off from IBI on his sixth birthday. I can't tell you how important IBI is for my son. He has made tremendous strides. It's the only intervention that gives us hope for a brighter future. To cut him off now is like pushing him off a cliff without a parachute. Actually...it feels like you're pushing my entire family off a cliff," I said, standing strong.

She didn't respond but let me continue.

"As a family, we're all affected by his progress. This is a fall that my family and I might never recover from. I'm asking—begging—you and your team to please, *please* not cut my son off from these services. This is the equivalent of chemo treatment and his chance of having a productive life."

I knew my time was ticking away, with just a few minutes left, as her wet hands were almost dry. I willed her to see the desperation in my glossy eyes and my sincere raw emotion. She reciprocated the focused attention as she wiped her hands with a paper towel.

"I understand what you're saying. We *are* listening to parents and are going to do whatever we can to make sure your son and all the other children with autism receive the services they need." Her voice bounced off the wall tiles.

I wanted so desperately to believe her, but I needed confirmation. I approached her, getting as close as I could without seeming confrontational, and put a tremendous amount of tenderness and compassion in my voice. "Please, I beg of you: make sure my baby boy is not forgotten. Please don't forget me. I'm a mother who's at your mercy."

I wasn't sure whether it was an act or whether I actually got to her, but a tear made a path down her face.

Since she didn't move, I continued. "You have the power to make a difference in our lives—make it matter," I said, releasing my pressed-together praying hands to wipe a tear off my own cheek.

She continued to look straight into my eyes. With her clean, dry hands, she touched the side of my arm and said, "I am listening, and I will not forget you. I understand and will do whatever I can to help."

This genuine response finally made me believe her.

Three years after this incident, we would be one of the first families to have government IBI services reinstated.

Surprisingly, years later, John had a private conversation with her, and in that conversation, she brought up this very incident. In this moment, I had no idea that she would remember me vividly and be affected by my words.

We never know what effect our words and actions will have.

THIRTY-THREE

A Father's Release

Exhausted.

My endless advocating, along with teaching, would be enough to make anyone long for a good night's sleep, but my sleep was still being controlled by Giaci's.

Giaci's room was a calm environment, with warm, subdued colours to reduce sensory stimuli. Despite this, he'd fall asleep for a couple of hours and then awaken, restless and eager to get moving. It was as if he had an internal alarm clock that would wake him at two or three a.m. Not all autistic persons have sleep issues, but Giaci absolutely did. He could function on little to no sleep, and every time he woke, he'd greet us with a smile on his bright little face.

Night after night he would wake up laughing hysterically, as if he were listening to his own private comedy show. He would go downstairs and raid the kitchen, eating everything he could since no one was there to stop him. Then he'd run around the house, turn on all the lights, and blast the volume on the television.

His sleep habits wreaked havoc on John and me, leaving us exhausted before our days even started. We tried every tip we found to help him sleep through the night: melatonin, relaxation techniques before bed, warm baths, consistent bedtime routines—you name it, we tried it. I refused to medicate him, though, for fear of other issues, like addiction or side effects.

One night, I awoke to rambunctious party sounds and laughter echoing against the high ceiling. I forced myself out of bed to hunt down our party animal and found the house lit up like the Las Vegas strip. The twins' bedroom door was wide open, and I could hear the Cartoon Network channel blaring on the television. As I approached their daisy-patterned walls at the entrance of their bedroom, I felt a breeze and smelled the scent of lavender plug-ins.

When I turned into their room, I was struck by the sight of my little boy standing on the queen-sized bed, between the twins' sleeping bodies.

The ceiling fan was on its highest speed—the source of the breeze I'd felt—and the movement of the blades created shadows of muted hues, softening the view of Giaci pouring a glass of water over the girls; despite all this, they still didn't wake up.

As soon as he caught a glimpse of me, he flopped down, sandwiched in between the girls. I approached with caution; it was hard not to smile at seeing my little hotdog smooshed between two slices of bread like this. He had the biggest smile plastered on his face, revealing that he wasn't asleep, though his eyes were closed in imitation of his sisters. Through it all, the girls were comatose.

A vein in my forehead pulsed as I hovered over his frozen smirk.

"Giaci," I said in a low, guttural voice, "go to your room right now!" I pointed in the direction of his room. His eyes fluttered open, and he saw me steaming. He knew I meant business. He leaped out of the bed and darted out, but I knew he wouldn't head straight for his room. I followed him, quietly rumbling, "No, to bed!"

Wide awake now, I followed Giaci as he Tigger-jumped down the hallway, avoiding his room until the last possible second. With a playful smile, he jumped into his bed. I gave him a final glare and shut his door.

Before going back to my bedroom, I went around the house, returning everything to its pre-party state, shutting off lights and the two televisions and closing the fridge door. Then I tried unsuccessfully to get a few hours of sleep.

When we got up in the morning, the first to appear downstairs was the happy-go-lucky Giaci. He descended the stairs in high spirits, as if he'd just had the fullest, best sleep of his life. Clearly he was created to be the life of the party. John and I just looked at each other and shook our heads in disbelief; there were no signs of him being tired at all.

Soon after, the twins and Lauren came down. We thought they'd surely be droopy-eyed and on Team Tired with us. Not so. They sat down at the table, all looking well rested.

As Carolina began eating her cereal, she pushed up her glasses and turned to me to ask, "Mommy, Giaci slept really good last night, didn't he? We didn't hear him at all!"

I turned to the other four-year-old and saw Maria nodding enthusiastically in agreement. "Giaci! You slept so good!" Maria patted Giaci on his back, appearing to approve of the previous night's behaviour.

I looked over at John, and we nearly burst out laughing. "Yes, honey, he sure did. He sure did," I said, winking at John.

"Never a dull moment in our house, right, my love?" John came over to wrap his arms around us all. It was hard to stay angry, no matter how unbelievably tired we both were. John was right: at least it was never boring in our home.

* * *

Despite how tired we were, the next day after school, John and I still had to meet with school staff for an Identification, Placement, and Review Committee (IPRC) meeting for our son. This meeting was to discuss Giaci's individual education plan (IEP) and his placement for the following year.

Lauren and Giaci attended the school where I taught for a few reasons: I thought the school was stellar, and not just because I was one of the teachers; it was located in a safe and secure neighbourhood; it was much easier for me to take the kids to school, which decreased my travel time; and I was able to see Giaci more at school. It was difficult for me to detach myself from him, as my mania for keeping him close chimed in my head constantly. But the school staff had been telling me about a more specialized classroom at another school days before this meeting. I anticipated more specifics would be given at this meeting, so John and I both made ourselves available and had his mom watch the twins while my mom took Giaci and Lauren.

John and I walked into the school as a united front. I had an annoying nervous tickle in my throat. I understood this school system and knew that the staff had little experience teaching children with autism. The teacher still didn't know how to apply ABA or any specialized behavioural interventions into his school days. The educational assistant tried her best, but she too was not trained in behavioural intervention. Making me even more nervous was the fact that these were my colleagues we were meeting with. I felt exposed. Plus, Giaci was being assessed by those who didn't know him the way I did, people who were falling back on their preconceived notions based on their inexperience with autism.

We walked into the meeting room and were greeted by knowing gazes. Parent-staff meetings were sometimes uncomfortable, but this was a new level of awkwardness. I felt a bit vulnerable as we said hello to the five women sitting opposite us: the principal, the learning support teacher, the classroom teacher, the educational assistant, and the special education advisor.

It was intimidating being outnumbered, and the tension was evident on both sides. No one knew how this was going to pan out. All the staff had paperwork arranged in front of them as if they were marking their territory, while John and I came empty-handed and open-hearted.

We all sat motionless until the principal, Catia, began the meeting.

"Thank you all for coming today. We are going to discuss Giaci's progress and where we think he ought to be placed in the next school year."

John and I watched her with attentive eyes.

Next, Mrs. Joan, the classroom teacher, began to go over her classroom observations.

I repositioned myself in my chair, trying to prepare for what came next.

Mrs. Joan started out strong. She wanted us to know that Giaci was loved and that she admired his rambunctious energy. After complimenting him, though, she jumped into a performance review. "He has a hard time following instruction, and he doesn't participate in circle time with the others." She explained everything we already knew about Giaci: that he was a runner, that he wanted to get away from the educational assistant whenever he could, and that, with his minimal language, he didn't interact with his peers.

Once she got started, the bleak report kept going and going, smacking us in the face. We had to keep our composure and hide the blows to our egos. It's not that John and I were surprised—we knew all of these things about Giaci—but it was quite another thing to hear everything "wrong" about our son in front of a crowd.

"Giaci is holding a pencil, and we're starting to write letters to form his name, but he needs a lot of support to do this," she said, keeping her focus on our faces.

After the teacher and educational assistant had recounted their evaluation of my son's educational profile, the principal and the learning support teacher spoke about his placement for the coming school year.

"After reviewing Giaci's progress, we would like to recommend that he attend Shoreline Elementary in a specialized education classroom. We have loved having him here but feel he would be better served in a classroom that has fewer students and where the teacher–pupil ratio is one to eight."

"So, for every eight students there will be a special education teacher and possibly three other support staff," said the learning support teacher.

The principal kept her eye on our reactions and then said, "Rita and

John, we want what is best for your son and feel that he would be better served at Shoreline Elementary."

My separation anxiety spiked. How would I be able to see him if he were at another school? How would I know what was happening to him? Giaci couldn't recount his days to me like the girls could, so we'd be left even more in the dark about his days at school.

"Giaci has so much more in him that has not been tapped into yet," I finally chimed in. "All I've heard tonight are the things that he *can't* do. But we're seeing progress with him at home, so why isn't this being seen at school?" I waited a beat before declaring, "I'm not comfortable with him being sent somewhere else."

I felt strong in my assertion, but all I saw in the other women's eyes was pity. These were the looks I'd always tried to avoid, the looks of *Poor Rita—she hasn't accepted her son's limitations.*

John sat as if he were sedated. This was the first time he'd been in the room when a professional discussed Giaci's academics and behaviours at school. I was used to these meetings, but John wasn't.

"Giaci just learns differently, and everything I've read indicates that ABA or IBI is what he needs. Why can't this be implemented at school? It's simply a different method of teaching. This is what my son needs to improve his life." I pleaded my case. It sounded like a script, but fuelling the words was the belief I had in them. It hadn't failed me yet.

The group stared at me, knowing full well that the school board did not have enough knowledge and experience with ABA or IBI to implement it. Training for staff was not being conducted at this time.

To divert the conversation, Catia asked, "Mr. Miceli, what are your thoughts?"

John responded with dead silence. My eyes shifted from the five women to my husband. At this point, all eyes were on him. He sat with his face lowered, staring at the floor as if a pause button had been pushed on him. Then, I heard him release a familiar sound:

"Ahem."

More silence followed.

No one else would have recognized what this sound meant: that he was focused on maintaining his demeanour. I alone knew what was coming: John was going to lose his composure.

"Okay! This meeting is over." I frantically waved my hands and tried to guide John to a standing position. I was interrupted by John's deep abdominal breath. I quickly motioned for the other women to leave, but they were confused by my abrupt behaviour.

We didn't even get to the door before John let out a childlike whimper. The women were stunned as John let his guard down, showing a father's tender heart. Tears of pain flowed onto his chiselled cheeks as he released years of pent-up hurt.

I turned to the principal, Catia, waving the white flag of defeat through my gaze. She gestured for the others to leave as I stood in front of John, obstructing his outburst from their view. I gently placed my hand on his curved back, rubbing back and forth, hoping to provide comfort with my touch.

"I know. I know." My eyes welled with tears of my own as the tables turned. John had finally broken. I wasn't the one crying this time; he was. I stood in front of him, up close, eye to eye as he was sitting in the chair. Our foreheads touched.

"We'll be okay. Giaci will be okay. We've got this." I tried to muster all my John-like bravado for him. For a moment, I understood all those times when he'd consoled me. He had to keep it together for us. And now, it was my turn to keep it together for him.

The principal gave us a moment to compose ourselves. She stood motionless and glossy-eyed at the far end of the room, blocking the door to prevent any interruptions.

After a few minutes, I turned to her and said, "We'll have to continue this another day," before turning back to John.

He was still trying to gather himself, unable to quiet the sniffling sounds. Catia took a step closer, as if she wanted to say something comforting but knew there was nothing left to say. She also knew that we couldn't take any more. Then John stood up, shrugged off the embarrassing incident as if it were a slight chill, and said goodbye.

My heart ached for my husband. Normally, everyone saw a strapping thirty-one-year-old man who exuded brawniness, confidence, and intelligence. They never expected him to expose a raw, feeble, private side of himself. John had just exposed his beating heart, but it wasn't a sign of weakness; it was a testament to the strength of a father who carried the pain of the child he adored.

* * *

The next day at school was even more uncomfortable for me. Most of these women had a hard time facing me, as I did them. We crossed paths in the hallway, trying to not make eye contact while still maintaining our professionalism.

I wanted to forget that the previous day had even happened, but I couldn't. The message that they wanted Giaci to go to another school was out in the open now; there was no hiding how they all felt. Throughout the day, I was consumed with wondering whether changing schools was the right choice for Giaci. I couldn't think about myself or how difficult it would be to be away from him. My maternal intuition was sounding an alarm again, and I couldn't snooze it for the sake of comfort.

At the end of the day, I entered Catia's office and asked to visit the specialized classroom at the other school.

"As difficult as this is for us, we need to make sure that our son's needs are being met," I said with as much conviction as I was able to muster.

She looked up from her desk and gave me a soft, understanding nod.

"I couldn't agree more. I'm confident that you'll see this classroom is a better fit. Talk to the teacher and the support staff. Ask as many questions as you can to put your mind at ease."

* * *

It wasn't easy to let go of control, but after visiting the specialized classroom, I made a list of the pros and cons. The cons all revolved around me not seeing him at my school. I had to stop trying to control everything and trust in the staff that had the knowledge and experience that I was looking for. John and I decided that for the next school year, when Giaci was almost seven, he would go to this new school, where they were trained in behavioural intervention.

Once Giaci did start at Shoreline Elementary, his new teacher, Ms. Lindsay, was able to put a stop to his "running away" behaviours and formed a bond of trust with our son. With time, Giaci began writing sentences and reading simple books. His language skills slowly increased. We made the right decision sending him there, and all it had taken was letting go.

THIRTY-FOUR

"Normal" Family Activities

When friends at work talked about their family trips or outings, I envied how seamless and easy their lives sounded. "Ordinary" family activities were not ordinary for us. We were used to half-watched movies at the theatre because of the disruptive noises that Giaci made, and spontaneously going out for dinner meant Giaci throwing a tantrum and us leaving before we had even finished the meal.

To mitigate this, we stopped trying to do "normal" family activities. We had to create our own version of normalcy in our family's everyday existence. We tried to set up a movie-theatre-feel and watched movies at home. If we were planning on eating out, we made sure we knew it would be a slow night at the restaurant.

With everything going well at Giaci's new school and him adjusting better to new experiences, I thought it was time to bring a new adventure to our family. I wanted the girls to have typical family experiences, and I was prepared to do whatever it took to make that happen.

One night, after the kids were all in bed and John and I were cozied up, enjoying our alone time watching reruns on TV, I turned to him with childlike eyes.

"John, what do you think about going on a family vacation?" I bounced on the couch cushion awaiting his response.

It came immediately. "Ri! Let's do Disney World in Florida!" He joined me in my childish bouncing; John was a huge fan of anything Disney, and so was Giaci.

"I know he loves Disney movies," I said, "but do you think we can do it? It would be a lot…"

John urged me out of my hesitation.

"I think we have to try! Besides, you never know unless we do." The affirmation in his voice made me a believer.

The next day I made the arrangements. Even though we knew it would be scorching, August was the only month John and I could get away from our work schedules. I knew that we would have to prepare Giaci for this week-long trip filled with new surroundings and an interruption to his routine. When he was younger, he hadn't been fazed by changes in his environment; I could take him anywhere and it didn't bother him in the least. However, now, at seven years old, his awareness of the world around him had increased, and he became easily distressed by any shifts in his everyday life or anything out of his routine. At school, the daily schedule had to be followed exactly or he would get upset and not comply. He would not participate if instead of a scheduled gym class there was an art lesson. He would still try to go to the gym to get what he wanted. Routine was mandatory in his world; it was crucial for holding off his anxiety. An anxiety explosion would look like him protesting with a loud "NO" or an escape to the bathroom. Any type of excursion had to be planned, then practised.

He always had to sit in the same seat in the minivan, right behind me. If one of his sisters sat in his spot, he would sit on top of them until they moved. He knew the exact routes to our usual destinations, and if I swerved away from the familiar path, he would protest from the back seat.

"Turn right, Mommy," I'd hear. "This way, Mommy!" He'd raise his little index finger like he was the conductor of an orchestra. Everything had to be the way he wanted it, the way he expected it, the predictable way he knew.

An adventure to the Magic Kingdom could turn his world upside down, but we had to try. For the girls. For John and me. Even for Giaci, because we knew the minute he saw the pool at the hotel and all the Disney magic, he would love it.

A plan of action was needed to get him there. We would have to teach Giaci a multitude of steps to help him anticipate and adjust to this new experience, and the reward at the end—time in the pool—had to be clearly communicated. He loved swimming, and for Giaci, that would be something worth working for. We needed to tackle this the way we did everything else: one step at a time.

In March, we began addressing Giaci's high anxiety with airports and airplanes, months prior to our August trip. Many people have a fear of planes and airports, but for Giaci it would result in aggressive and noncompliant behaviour. When he was little and we went to New York, he didn't understand planes, so this fear wasn't present. For some reason, this fear had developed as he grew and learned more. We'd noticed it when we went on a trip to Arizona to visit family. Giaci's anxiety was the highest I'd ever seen it, and he had a few meltdowns. His fear of the airport and airplanes was clearly shown, and we really struggled to get him home. We didn't want this trip to be like that one.

We began by showing him a video of the boarding process. He responded with, "No! No thank you!" He raised his eyebrows, and there was anguish in his eyes. The video showed a family walking into an airport, boarding the airplane, greeting the flight attendants, and being seated on the plane. We kept showing him the video, and his comfort level increased after a few weeks because he was still safe on the ground. We took data on his reaction, noting his level of stress, facial expression, and verbal responses. When he seemed comfortable watching these videos, we knew it was time to step up the sensory experience.

Next, we started driving to the local airport with Megan and Kelly, his behaviour therapists. This airport was much smaller than the airport we would be departing from, much closer, and much easier to navigate for this particular exercise. I asked John to call the airport representatives ahead of time so they were aware of our activity. This was easy since he knew the chief executive officer of the airport, Phil. After their call, Phil informed his staff of what we would be doing and subsequently let us know that everyone was onboard and supportive.

"Rita, I called and spoke to Phil," said John. "He said we are more than welcome to practise with Giaci at the airport. He has a picture of Giaci and has shown his staff so that they are aware. He also said his staff are more than happy to help with anything we need."

"That's awesome, John." It warmed my heart to have this level of acceptance and understanding.

We started making daily visits. After the third trip it became more difficult because Giaci knew exactly where we were going. He would frantically tell me which route to take so that we wouldn't go in the direction of the airport. "Mommy, turn left. Let's go home, Mommy," he repeated, hoping I would turn around. After parking the van, I took his hand to help him out, and his palms were soaked with sweat.

The first two visits involved us just sitting in the van outside the airport entrance doors.

"No, Mommy, NO! Let's go home right now," Giaci said.

"It's okay, Giaci. Kelly and Megan and Mommy will help you. Breathe, Giaci, you're okay." I used my most reassuring tone to coax him through. Nothing Kelly, Megan or I said seemed to help, so we took notes on his behaviour and reassured him as best we could.

"Tomorrow we'll go inside for a quick visit," I said one day, reassuring him that he would be safe.

The next day we did exactly that. Kelly was on one side of Giaci and I on the other, while Megan followed a few steps behind in case he ran back toward the van.

When he resisted, we grabbed him securely by the arms. "Giaci, we're just going to walk up to that pole and back," I pointed to show him that it was only a few steps, "and then we'll go back home. But first, we walk to that pole and back. Then home."

When he accomplished what we had asked, we praised him and never pushed him further. We wanted to make sure that Giaci trusted our word, so if we said, "Only to the pole and back," we made sure not to stretch our agreement.

We spent weeks inching him closer and closer to the airplane. In time, we saw that he was ready for the next push out of his predictable world.

Two weeks before our departure, Giaci watched me take out the suitcases. He immediately reverted to an anxiety-ridden state.

"No, no more." He wrung his hands together, squeezing his face with tension.

Any other requests made on him that day would be met with adamant opposition, so we didn't push any further. We let him adjust to seeing the suitcases.

Once he was comfortable seeing them in our home and showed us that he was more relaxed during our visits to the airport, it was time to go to the actual airport that we were departing from, which was close to an hour's drive away.

Giaci was not a fan of this change of scenery. My heart ached because I had to put him through these difficult experiences, but there was no other way. Kelly and Megan didn't speak the entire drive, to minimize any potential auditory sensory overload for Giaci.

Kelly sat with him in the backseat. She noticed that his palms were drenched in sweat from the moment we left the house to when we parked the car. Once again, we surrounded him with loving security and began our reassurance.

"It's okay, buddy! We're just going to walk around the airport and then go home!" Kelly said.

"It's time to go home," he said, glaring at me.

When he didn't hear what he wanted to hear, his body remained tight and wound up, but eventually he made it inside and back out again. The second he reached his goal, we jumped back into the van, and I said, "See? We're going home right now, buddy!" and took a big breath with him. Another box checked off our list.

The ride home was wordless and easier on Giaci. He seemed emotionally depleted and too exhausted to say or do anything.

When we arrived home, Kelly and Megan's shift ended, and Giaci walked to his bedroom rubbing his eyes and calling it a night.

I too was drained but needed to talk to John and the girls about getting their help. They were going to play a fundamental role in this plan. Giaci, his therapists and I had laid the groundwork. Now I needed John and the girls to be ready to take their places.

As we sat on the couch in the living room, I detailed the strategic plan,

"Okay, family, we have to remember not to talk a lot because that makes Giaci more agitated. Minimal words to keep him as calm as possible. The bags will be put in the van when Giaci is sleeping, so we'll have breakfast like always and then get in the van as if it were a normal day." I spoke clearly, and all eyes were focused on me.

"We cannot take our eyes off Giaci once we get to the airport. We have to all grab our bags and surround him constantly so we can help him through this and have a great Disney vacation." I felt like a coach pumping up my players in a team huddle.

Upon hearing the plan, their game faces emerged. Never did I sense resentment or frustration; their focus was filled with the purest love.

Maria took on the role of spokesperson for her two sisters. "For sure, Mommy. We're ready."

I finished my talk with, "Okay, girls, we can do this! I know how much you love your brother, so let's do this and make great memories."

Carolina and Maria jumped off the couch and nodded in agreement.

Lauren stood up straight and said, "We've got this," before they all went off to their rooms to get ready for bed.

* * *

When departure day came, my hands trembled, but I had to maintain my composure so as not to alarm anyone, especially Giaci. We started the day with our typical wake-up, breakfast, and clean-up routine. I had strategically placed the suitcases in the back of the van the night before, so they were not in Giaci's sight. I figured it was one less thing for him to have to process and perseverate over.

When it was time to leave, I kept it casual, as if we were just going for a family drive.

"Time to go, everybody!" I said. "Let's get in the van."

We all assembled, and Giaci followed our lead, as this was not out of the ordinary. However, once we went in an unfamiliar direction, he clued in on the situation and began issuing his backseat driver directives. "Daddy, turn left. Go this way," he commanded. "It's time to go home, Daddy," he kept repeating.

When we parked the van at the airport, there was immediate fear in his eyes. His body tensed just like it had during the practice round, but our family was ready.

We moved as a pack, surrounding him like bodyguards around a superstar. We each grabbed a suitcase with one hand and kept the other hand free to hold onto Giaci or be ready to grab him if we had to. I had all our documents ready to show the Customs and Border Protection officer while my family kept Giaci safe and occupied with his Disney videos and earphones.

Once we had put our carry-on bags on the conveyor belt, we each had to cross through the scanner. I made sure to have the doctor's note stating Giaci's diagnosis ready for the officer, who nodded and let me wait for Giaci on the other side. We were so close to our goal that we could all taste it. We watched Giaci walk through the scanner with ease. Now, all that was left was waiting to board at our assigned gate.

I had snacks, an iPad, his VTech toy, earphones, calming nutritional supplements, and visual aids to help Giaci process what was going to happen. Each photo was placed in order on a strip of cardboard with Velcro. The first picture was of our family in the van. Then, there was a picture of the airport. The next was of an airplane, and the last one was of Giaci in a swimming pool with a ginormous smile on his face. The visuals helped reduce his anxiety because they showed him what was going to happen next. As we waited, he glanced at the visual cues, and then through the window at the airport, trying his best to remember everything he had been taught over the past few months.

Before boarding began, I approached the counter to speak to the attendant, who was focused on her computer screen.

"Hi there!" I smiled, hoping to ease her into our situation. "My son has autism, and he gets very nervous about flying. Would you possibly allow us to board the plane first so we can get him settled before we fly? We really want to start our first Disney vacation on the right foot." I spoke with every ounce of sincerity I had as I held out his doctor's note.

The attendant lowered her glasses and looked up at me.

"Hello, my dear! You'll be able to board first," she said. "And you don't need to show me your note. Just stand in that line." She winked and then pointed in the direction I needed to go.

I thanked her and walked back toward John, who was guarding Giaci. Our strategy was to keep Giaci as calm as possible before the culminating moment of boarding the plane.

As I stood in the assigned line for elderly people and young children, I noticed an older woman in a wheelchair behind me. She was frail but talkative and was with a woman who resembled her but looked half her age; I assumed it was her daughter. I could feel the older woman glaring my way, clearly not understanding why I was in this line in the first place, let alone in front of her.

She spoke to her daughter loud enough so that I could hear:

"This line is for the *elderly* and *young children*. Why is she here? She shouldn't be here." She rambled until her daughter shushed her.

I was tempted to turn around and explain my situation but was too stressed to exert any additional effort. I was too close to the already emotional climax. I kept my back to her and continued to tap my feet, waiting for the flight attendant to allow us to proceed. John was still holding Giaci tight in the sitting area as he and the girls waited for my signal.

When the time arrived to board the plane, the flight attendant nodded to me, which set off a chain reaction. I turned to wave to John, he turned to whisper to the girls, and they then darted into action. Without speaking, they grabbed their bags and filled in the gaps around Giaci.

They were a unit that marched tightly in unison surrounding Giaci like a defensive shield. They joined me in line. We were so close!

When we approached the doorway to advance toward the plane, I knew what was going to happen before it did. Giaci's face became tight, and his eyes opened wide. He tried pushing and pulling his way free of us and was loudly saying "NO, no plane! Mommy, no plane!" The Tasmanian devil erupted in him, causing a scene. He became aggressive and flailed a free hand and one foot, squirming to be set free. He got louder with an ear-splitting shriek and yelled, "No, no airplane!" with conviction. We stayed the course and continued to move our family unit forward.

The girls were accustomed to ignoring onlookers, and they knew we just needed to keep moving in the direction of the plane. We had to keep our eye on the finish line. John and I, with a stiff, firm hold on Giaci, ignored his verbal and physical protest, and forged ahead.

As this scene exploded, I glanced sideways at the older woman who had been grumbling under her breath just moments before. She had stopped talking and now sat dumbfounded as she watched us board before her. She understood now. Part of me still wanted to turn to her and explain, "See? This is why!" but it wasn't worth my energy. I had more pressing matters to focus on, like getting Giaci onto that plane and into his seat.

As we walked down the boarding bridge, we continued to hang onto him with a strong grip.

"Almost there, Giaci, almost there. First airplane and then swimming. You can do it Giaci. You can do it." I said softly and calmly. The final tool in our arsenal was the promise of swimming. After having put him through this ultimate stressful experience, we had to reward him with what he loved. I had packed his bathing suit in his backpack, which I had securely strapped to my shoulder. We would be ready to let him go swimming as soon as we arrived at our hotel.

As we approached the plane, the scene was much more familiar to him because of all the boarding simulation videos we had shown him for weeks. Still, as we neared our seats, Giaci clamped onto my hair with all his force. It was a last-ditch effort to protest this activity, and I was the casualty of this attack. He pulled on my hair so powerfully that I thought there would be a hole in the back of my scalp.

John couldn't get Giaci to release his fierce grip, so I clamped onto my hair with my two hands to try to release his fingers. The stewardess approached our battle scene and stood frozen, shaken by our actions.

Finally, John was able to forcibly free me from Giaci's hold and plunked him down into his seat. John was breathing heavily, the girls were mortified and stressed, and I ached with pain, but we'd made it.

We belted Giaci in between me and John so he'd have nowhere to go for the duration of the flight. Sitting between us, he slumped and grumbled like subdued thunder. My hands were trembling as I tried to adjust my own seatbelt and smooth out my hair. John leaned over behind Giaci to see how I was.

"I'm sorry, honey. Are you hurt?" he asked.

Unable to speak, I shook my head no, while focusing most of my energy on not crying. We'd caused enough of a scene for one day. My head throbbed where Giaci had pulled a chunk of hair out, but my suffering inside was far greater. I hoped this all would be worth it.

By the time the rest of the passengers began to board, I'd managed to compose myself and carry on as if nothing had happened. Giaci didn't make a fuss in his seat now; he sat quietly. From my son's backpack, I pulled out activities for him. He normally enjoyed watching videos on his iPad, eating potato chips, and squeezing his squishy ball. I also pulled out the visual strip. I showed him the pictures and explained the day's events once again in a soothing, yet firm voice.

"Giaci, look! First our family was in the van," I said as I lifted this picture off the Velcro. It made a distinctive ripping sound. I put the little square picture of our family in the van in a plastic bag I had ready.

"That's all done! Next, we went to the airport," I said, pointing to the airport picture on the strip. I peeled this picture off as well and put this in the plastic bag too.

"That is all done. Now we're on the airplane." I pointed to the airplane picture.

"See, Giaci! We are on the airplane." I hoped the confusion in his mind had settled down so that he could process the information.

"And you know what's next, buddy? Swimming! After the airplane, we're going swimming!"

When he responded, his voice was deflated but he confirmed the plan.

"Mommy, first plane, then swimming." His upturned eyes begged me to make this happen sooner rather than later.

"Yes, buddy. First airplane and then swimming," I responded.

He seemed momentarily satisfied with this answer, but he was still uneasy about being on the plane. Occasionally, he would curiously peer out the airplane window. Seeing nothing but unfamiliarity, he would slam the window shade shut. He repeatedly opened and closed the window shade the entire flight while mumbling, "Mommy, first airplane, then swimming." He would follow that by getting right in my face. His eyes were almost touching my eyes. He wanted to make sure I was listening to his proclamation. I pulled his bathing suit out of his backpack to verify that this was going to happen.

John and the girls put on their earphones to try to find their happy places, knowing full well that the stress would pass. That left me with Giaci and a plane full of people peeking over at us with curiosity. I could only imagine what the other passengers were thinking as our conversation repeated over and over again for all to hear.

The end was near, and even I was ready to get off the plane by the time the pilot announced our descent into Florida.

"Almost there, buddy. We're almost done," I reiterated, using the vocabulary that was familiar to him, trying to calm his restlessness.

Once we had landed and the aircraft came to a complete stop, I finally saw a glimpse of repose on Giaci's adorable little face. His eyes were not as tight, and the corners of his mouth turned up.

As we stood, waiting for our turn to walk down the aisle and off the plane, an older gentleman turned to face us. "I'll bet you're going swimming after this," he said with a smile directed at Giaci.

I let out a sigh of relief; he clearly understood our situation. Knowing that Giaci wasn't able to answer him and was too preoccupied with getting off the plane as soon as possible, I smiled and answered, "Yes, that's exactly where we're going. How did you know?"

Safe on the ground, Giaci seemed more at ease. Still, the girls, John, and I continued to surround him with a circle of soothing comfort. I couldn't believe that we were fulfilling the family game plan. We were moments away from a family trip to Disney World! No matter what happened beyond these doors, we had made it here, and that was enough for me.

THIRTY-FIVE

Disney Bliss

Even the shuttle ride to Disney was magical.

Giaci was preoccupied by the cartoon playing on the TV screen in front of him, and for a moment he forgot we were even going swimming. Giaci loved all things Disney, and the fact that the entire bus was decorated from top to bottom with the characters he knew kept him sitting calmly next to me.

Disney made our family delirious with joy. We all had the same contagious smile that had graced Giaci's face, and the girls were wide-eyed as they took in all the Disney characters on the bus and on the screens. John and I were warmed by their excitement and eager to start our first family vacation.

As soon as we pulled into the All-Star Movies Resort, Giaci remembered our agreement and tugged on John to take him to the pool. John looked at me like a kid asking for permission to wander off.

I laughed at John's inner child coming out to play and said, "We're on vacation! Let's do whatever we want."

John beamed at my nod, looking as excited as Giaci was to get right into the Disney action. The girls couldn't hide their eager faces either, so I shooed them away to put their bathing suits on in the lobby bathrooms while I got us all checked in.

After I had gotten our room keys and left our luggage at the front desk, I went to check on my family in the pool area. You couldn't miss the water bouncing off Giaci, who was smiling brighter than the Florida sun. The girls were sitting at the edge of the pool with John, and they were all watching Giaci. He was captivating when he was this energetic, erupting with squeaking sounds of sheer euphoria.

I smiled and waved at my beautiful family as I approached them, already feeling like all our hard work and preparation had been worth it. The feeling of the sun on our skin was enough to relax us; I hardly recognized us anymore. We'd all come so far. There was no tension in our eyes, no thoughts about pushing more language or having to do more, be more. We were in a magical moment, an uncomplicated dreamy world, innocent and carefree. We were soaking it all in.

Was this what our life could be like? I thought about what it had taken to get Giaci here, but we had done it, and we could keep doing it. We were a team, a force to be reckoned with. Together we could do anything.

I placed a hand on John's shoulder and gave it a good squeeze. He looked up at me with that same childlike smile as if to say *We did it!* Then he splashed me with his foot. Giaci didn't leave the water, the girls didn't leave Giaci's side, and John and I just didn't want to leave the magic we'd found at Disney World. This was paradise, and we'd created it ourselves.

* * *

We spent the evening settling in for our week in Disney and enjoyed dinner at our hotel's food court. Disney made even food courts seem magical! Around every corner there were movie characters and scenes to take in. However, watching how the girls interacted with Giaci was the most magical experience of all.

Lauren was the enforcer, always trying to stretch him to more independence. "Come on, Giaci, let's go get our food. Pick up this tray and come with me." She pointed to the tray. "Good, Giaci! Watch me. Watch Lauren." She then guided him to where he had to go in the buffet line. She had modelled actions for him many times before and was by now a seasoned expert.

Carolina and Maria, on the other hand, excelled in the "fun sisters" department. Carolina in particular knew exactly how to get Giaci's attention by moving right into his field of vision. She would move in close enough that he couldn't be distracted by other things around him, and he practically *had* to lay eyes on her.

The three girls made every educational moment fun-filled, and they never seemed stressed out when it came to their brother. They were motivated to help him feel good because it meant we would all feel good.

Sitting down to eat was always easy with Giaci. Food was his motivator and true love, but the hard part was getting him to walk away from the buffet. Even though we were on vacation, we wanted to make sure he was eating well and maintaining a level of structure so he wouldn't feel sick or weighed down. While we weren't as strict with his diet as we once had been—we'd settled on something far more sustainable—we did continue to follow his vitamin supplements regimen, under the direction of his naturopathic doctor.

Thankfully, he was so wiped out from swimming and from all the delicious food that we were able to navigate him back to our room to get him rested for the busy day ahead.

* * *

The next morning, we were booked to have breakfast at the Grand Floridian Resort with Disney characters. We weren't sure how to explain this to Giaci, as it would be impossible, so we left it to surprise. Lauren, Maria, and Carolina were well aware of where we were going, and they were almost more excited to see how their brother would react than I was.

Giaci had always been an avid Disney movie watcher; in fact, you could say he was a fanatic! He could watch Disney movies dozens of times and never be bored. He had memorized most of them and would always smile just before his favourite parts came up. He loved knowing exactly what was going to happen and would even repeat lines from the movie.

We took the shuttle over to the Grand Floridian in the early morning. It was already steamy outside. Prepped with a day's worth of gear in our backpacks, we embarked on a day unlike any other. Giaci was going to watch his favourite characters come to life.

As soon as we arrived, we were escorted to our table by the hostess, who was dressed in a warm yellow dress with poofy sleeves and a white apron over it. "Welcome to your Supercalifragilistic Breakfast. Please follow me!" She beamed at us from beneath her floppy chef's hat.

As we followed her down the rows of restaurant tables, we were surrounded by a bright Disney soundtrack. I looked down at Giaci, who was giddy and bobbing along to the tune of "Bear Necessities," and then back at John and the girls, who were simply hungry and scurrying along. The smell of warm syrup and eggs wafted through the air, encouraging us to get to our seats faster. But before we could sit down, I heard a familiar squeak of excitement from Giaci. He had caught a glimpse of Tigger and Pooh from afar and was now jumping up and down, mimicking a Tigger spring.

"John! Look at him," I said as I tugged on the girls to wait. The hostess must have been used to these kinds of reactions because she looked just as peaceful as she had when greeting us. The girls began jumping up and down along with Giaci.

"Way to go, Giaci," Maria cheered.

"Jump, Giaci! Jump with Tigger!" Carolina added.

Giaci couldn't contain himself. He was bursting with an enchanted energy. We all followed Giaci toward Tigger and Winnie the Pooh, trying to catch up to him as he hopped along quickly. Tigger noticed Giaci's mighty hops and turned his energy toward him, which was the best-case scenario for Giaci. Besides "King Giaci," "Tigger" was our secondary nickname for him.

"Give Tigger a big hug, buddy!" John said, encouraging Giaci to feel the realness of this once-imaginary character.

Giaci leaped onto Tigger's giant legs, which made our hearts leap too. Pooh Bear looked sad to be left out, so Lauren encouraged Giaci to share the love, but he was too preoccupied with his favourite.

Our hearts were full of joy, and the rumbly in our tummies had to wait for the dreamy experience to fade. We weren't sure it ever would or that we even wanted it to. Giaci certainly didn't.

Still, we were hungry, so after a few minutes, John placed his hand on Giaci's shoulder and said, "Come on, Giaci, time to eat breakfast." John guided Giaci away from Tigger and toward our table without any sort of protest from Giaci, much to our surprise. He must have been hungry as well.

As scrumptious as the Mickey waffles were, Giaci kept his head turned toward the characters the entire time. I could only imagine what he was thinking; based on his expression, he was in complete awe of his hero. He was deliriously happy, laughing and smiling and taking it all in.

After breakfast, we made our way to the Magic Kingdom. The Disney energy was contagious, and characters followed us wherever we went. Every greeting was buoyant.

When Giaci saw Buzz Lightyear, he ran toward him and said "Buzz!" His face lit up like Buzz Lightyear's laser blast. The vivid colours shone off Cinderella Castle, capturing the girls' gaze as we approached it. Once inside, through the windows, golden sunbeams lit a path that guided us to Cinderella's Royal Table. The feast that awaited us smelled sweet like the aroma of banana bread. At the table, Giaci sat like a king, and smiled.

He was adapting well to the never-ending changes in his surroundings, probably because he recognized so many aspects of the park. Around every corner was a familiar face. No one would have guessed that he had autism. To the public we must have looked picture-perfect, just like the park, where you can't see all the work that goes into running the show. Here at Disney, we had checked our problems at the door and entered a magical world where everything and everyone was truly in the Happiest Place on Earth—including us.

Every day we encouraged new experiences for Giaci, and he was always rewarded with swimming in the afternoon. After the theme park, we would go back to our resort, and the kids would swim in the pool for hours as John and I lay back and watched. Our daughters took turns interacting with their brother in the water, foreshadowing the custodial women they would become. There was never resentment at having to watch over their brother; it came from an instinctual place of love.

We encouraged patience, understanding, and compassion to foster an unconditional love between them. The twins, who were two years younger than Giaci, acted like overprotective and overbearing sisters. The love they had for their brother was genuine and natural, planted in them from birth.

For my girls, having a brother with special needs added another layer to their characters. They possessed more empathy and compassion than most because they saw first-hand the struggles of living with autism. As long as I was around, I would make sure to tell them how amazing they were. It would have been impossible to go on this trip without them.

"We did a pretty good job, hey, John?" I nudged my lounging husband, who was reclined on a poolside chair.

He looked over at our splashing children and nodded.

"We sure did. Thank you for this," he said before leaning over and kissing me.

During the early years, it had been hard to see anything beautiful about our life, but my eyes were now open to the many precious moments that could be created while living with autism.

Our experience at Disney showed us what was possible when we worked together. It was our dream come true.

THIRTY-SIX

Fear of the Future

Now that Giaci was nine, I was becoming increasingly consumed with thoughts of the future. We saw slow and steady progress in the two previous years, but I knew now that he would never catch up to his peers. The gap just seemed to get larger and larger. Like most people, Giaci had good days and bad. On the good days, we showered each other with generous declarations of "I love you," along with hugs, smiles and kisses. The bad days, however, were always draining and sent me into a panic spiral. What would he be like when he got older? He would never be able to live completely on his own. These thoughts occupied a permanent space in my mind, and John and I soon began to talk about my concerns.

"Do you ever think about what Giaci will be like when he gets older?" I asked him one evening just before we settled down to watch an episode of *Family Feud*.

"Of course I do, but I can't think about it too much or it brings me down. We can't control the future. We can only deal with our present," he huffed before regaining his composure.

I knew that he hated ending the day with these conversations, but I just couldn't put it out of my mind.

"But who will take care of him when we aren't here? We know that someone is going to have to care for him full time," I said with certainty, though I knew I would never be satisfied with any answer. I didn't notice that spunky, seven-year-old Carolina was listening in from the kitchen until she spoke up:

"Mom, I'll take care of Giaci if something happens to you guys." She spoke with assertive positivity.

I turned to see her serious adult-like expression; if she had any doubts about her promise, it didn't linger on her face. She and her sisters thought they knew what it took to raise Giaci, and while they'd been doing a great job as siblings, there was quite a stretch from sibling to caregiver.

I sighed and collected my thoughts.

"That's beautiful, honey, but I don't want any of you girls to worry about your brother. You'll have your own lives to live. You'll be married and have families of your own one day! What if your future partner isn't interested in helping to care for your brother?" I suggested, thinking this would deter her.

Instead, Carolina sprinted across the room to stand right in front of me and John. She stuck her face close to ours.

"Mom. Dad. Listen!" Her caramel eyes didn't leave ours. She meant business. "First of all, I won't marry someone unless they love Giaci like I love Giaci." She kept her tone professional, as if she were pitching a business proposal. "Secondly, I love Giaci, and I *want* to take care of him. We've been doing it all this time, so why would we stop? I know Maria and Lauren feel the same way!"

She hadn't even finished her last sentence when my eyes began to water. The maturity and beauty of her response was incredibly powerful. It was a testament to her true character and an affirmation of a deeper level of love. It was proof that what I feared most had not happened. We could never be torn apart.

"I love you, honey, more than you could ever imagine," I said, grabbing a tissue to wipe away my tears. We hugged, and then she went upstairs to her room.

John didn't verbalize any sort of response, but his proud smile was a trifle smug, as if to say *I told you we didn't have to worry.*

He was right—we'd raised amazing kids.

* * *

The next morning, as we waited on the driveway for Giaci's school bus, the twins ran into the garage to grab a basketball. This was the daily routine: keep Giaci occupied so we wouldn't have to chase after him if he ran. He loved to run and get all his energy out, but at eight in the morning, the rest of us didn't have the same affinity for running around the block.

The girls and I made a circle in the driveway, and I manoeuvred Giaci into a spot beside me. Then, Maria bounce-passed the basketball over to Carolina and counted, "One," so that Giaci could hear and follow her lead.

Carolina caught the ball after it bounced in the centre of the circle and continued with the next number. "Two," she said, her eyes fixed on her brother, who was preparing himself to be next. The girls modelled the game so their brother could successfully participate and take his turn.

Since we had played this game many times before, he knew what the expectations were. It was now his turn, and as the ball bounced and travelled through the air in his direction, he raised his hands to receive it, smiling, and caught the ball. He then bounced it to Lauren and said "Three," while chuckling under his breath. He willingly participated in our game, and the counting continued until the bus arrived.

Once the bus was in sight, Carolina knew to put the ball back in the garage and to grab Giaci's backpack while Lauren and Maria stood guard. All I had to do was stand back and smile, watching the incredible connection between the four. It was a profound and uninhibited sibling bond.

When the bus stopped in front of our house, I reached for the special seatbelt harness that we used to fasten Giaci in on the bus. It was very constricting, with straps that completely surrounded his chest, and a back zipper with steel hooks to clamp onto the bus's seat. It reminded me of the straitjackets magicians donned and then freed themselves from to the overwhelming shock and amazement of spectators. Giaci often performed a similar act. We called him Houdini for a reason.

Before we got this seatbelt harness, Giaci would run up and down the aisle of the bus as it was moving. Having this additional harness prevented injury, but like Houdini, Giaci had managed to release himself from its constraints a few times. The bus driver and all the bus officials were in awe of his ability to manoeuvre his compact body, wiggling himself to freedom.

"How's Mr. Houdini over there?" the bus driver said in greeting as she swung open the doors.

I laughed and hoisted the seatbelt harness over my shoulder like a medal. "I've figured this thing out, and there's no way he's escaping on you today!"

Already sitting on the bus was Andrea, whose voice tumbled out of her the minute she laid eyes on us. "Hi, Giaci! Hi! Hi, Giaci! Hello!" She had fetal alcohol syndrome, which presented itself through antsy anxiety, keeping her talking incessantly.

Giaci was the opposite and typically needed prompting to respond, so I was the one who directed their brief conversation.

"Giaci, Andrea said hi! You need to answer," I said, slowing my speech, kneeling to his eye level, and pointing to Andrea.

"Hi," he said with narrowed eyes as he turned to the other side of the bus.

As Giaci settled in his spot, I wrapped the harness around his scrawny chest, zipping it up on the back side of his body. I then tugged the straps to their tightest setting to secure his safety. Last, I hooked the clamps to those on the seat, hoping for the safest ride to date.

"Love you, buddy," I said, kissing him on the forehead and knowing not to wait for a response. He was already trying to process too much sensory input, so for me to impose one more demand on him could only elevate his anxiety.

Giaci had to process the five senses of sight, sound, touch, smell and taste. He also had to process the vestibular sense, which is balance and sense of movement, and proprioception, which is the sense of knowing one's position in space. He had the visual brightness of the yellow school bus and the rising sun. He had the sound of the pulsating, rumbling engine. He had the sensation of touch with me gripping his hand and the weight of the harness over the core of his body. Then, there was the smell of the exhaust oozing out of the back pipe of the school bus and into his nostrils. There could have been other sensory effects coming at him that I wasn't even aware of.

There was so much for him to take in, and Giaci's brain managed information differently. The cords that linked his brain to his sensory system didn't send messages like mine or other neurotypical people's.

When we see something bright, our eyes automatically squint. Giaci's brain would mix up the message and instead tell his eyes to look intensely, so he'd feel the discomfort. With loud engine sounds, we would perhaps cover our ears with our hands, whereas Giaci would freeze and be overwhelmed by the most excruciating noise.

Under these conditions, his brain couldn't process a simple response of "Hi." It was impossible to know how all the sensory input was affecting him because he couldn't verbalize it. It was a guessing game.

For this reason, I always had to be in tune with his behaviour. There were certain facial expressions that only I could read, such as when he was getting sick. His eyes would glaze over, and he would take much longer than usual to answer. Paying attention to these slight changes in his behaviour helped me gauge the severity of the situation so I could respond appropriately.

Once I had secured my son in his seat, I said my goodbyes to Andrea and the bus driver and stepped off the bus. At this point, the girls were all in the van, ready to be taken to school. As I turned to watch the school bus drive away, I noticed Giaci giving himself his usual sensory fix, which involved pressing his face close to his hands and then squeezing them together as if he were twisting water out of a wet towel. He did this to help calibrate himself to his new environment and cope with his surroundings.

Once Giaci was out of sight, I got into my van and went to work. Teaching gave me a different sense of purpose; I had fun discovering these young personalities and was invested in shaping their futures much like I was with my own children. Teaching meant helping to create those light-bulb moments of discovery. I finally felt alert enough to be present for those moments and for all the other moments that make up a busy school day.

At home, I relied on a team of people to help Giaci with those same light-bulb moments. It had been more than three years since Giaci had been cut off from the government program at age six, but thanks to all our advocating and fighting, the IBI government program had started up for us again three months earlier. We now had access to a team of behaviour therapists overseen by a senior therapist and clinical psychologist, Dr. Barrera. Five days a week, an after-school behaviour therapist went down to the basement with Giaci to administer a two-hour therapy session.

Having the funded government program meant that John could work less, which allowed him to spend more time with the family. Having him home completed us; he was the link that kept us bound together.

However, coming home from one job led me straight into another: administrative assistant. The government gave us a choice of either the Direct Service Option (DSO) or the Direct Funding Option (DFO). We decided to go with the latter because even though it was more work for me to do the hiring, payroll, and paperwork submissions, I got to choose who was on our team and the direction of my son's learning.

After school, when we got home, and within minutes of me closing the garage door, the *ding-dong* chime rang from the front entrance. Before answering it, I grabbed a granola bar from the kitchen cupboard and handed it to Giaci to eat at the table. Right away he unwrapped it and took a monstrous bite while I went to let our team in.

Normally they'd all come at various times, but today I'd scheduled our monthly team meeting. Kelly and Megan had moved away to continue their educations, so we had two new therapists, Bella and Jamie, who were both university students, one in nursing and one in audiology.

Everyone greeted one another as they entered the foyer. Giaci had devoured his granola bar and was off and running down the basement stairs to where he would entertain himself on the computer. He moved like the Flash, his legs becoming one wheel as he zipped off. Knowing that Giaci was safe in the house, the team assembled at the kitchen table to discuss the data regarding his monthly progress.

The senior therapist, Karen, had come prepared with all her data arranged in manila file folders. She pulled them, as well as her laptop, out of her supersized tote bag and plunked them onto the granite table. She didn't live in our city but had a few clients in the area. For the entire hour, she pulled data up on her computer screen and directed the in-depth discussion of which steps Giaci was at in each task analysis.

The group discussions continued with recommendations and alterations to the programs if Giaci's progress was not advancing to a level of "mastery." An example of this was in learning to brush his teeth. He was first taught to unscrew the toothpaste cap. Once that step was mastered, he could move on to learning how to squeeze the tube and deposit toothpaste on the brush. To have "mastered" this skill, Giaci needed to be able to achieve 80 to 100 percent in two consecutive sessions with two different instructor therapists. He hadn't mastered this skill independently yet, but he would get there.

The skill also had to be generalized, which meant that he could apply a skill across all environments, with all people, and with different variations of that skill. For example, once he learned what a cup was, he had to be able to label the cup in a school, home, and restaurant; do so with a variety of family or friends; and label cups of different colours, sizes, and materials.

During the meeting, everyone had the opportunity to speak, including me, as I directed what my family and I believed was important for Giaci to learn, as well as the progress we observed. Every six months we had to submit an Individual Service Plan (ISP) to the government service provider for review, so it was crucial for us to meet consistently and update Giaci's work plan accordingly. We had to hit the Ministry benchmarks, which had been established by an expert clinical panel.

This panel recommended that benchmarks were necessary to monitor each child's progress and to ensure transparent clinical decision-making regarding the continuation of IBI. Otherwise, the discharge process would begin. Simply put, we had to hit specific expectations, or we would lose the government funding. It was a constant battle to hang on to these necessary services so Giaci could continue to learn skills that would eventually enable him to live as independently and productively as possible as he grew into a teenager and eventually into an adult.

Once the hour-long meeting was finished and our next meeting date was set, Bella went downstairs to work with Giaci, and the rest of the team left. There was no way any one of us could do this alone. We had to have this team approach. I was glad to have learned this because it would have been impossible to get him to where he was on my own. At one time, I tried to juggle all of this myself. Now I completely relied on my team of supporters, who were trained in behavioural strategies to help him acquire more and more skills.

One challenge for us was finding reliable therapists to employ. Since I could offer only minimal part-time hours, I mainly hired students. Having students meant that once they had finished their postgraduate schooling, they would move on to full-time employment elsewhere. Therapists cycled in and out of my home.

The hardest part of this arrangement was the emotional bond we'd develop with the people who came into our home daily. Many affected our lives, as Giaci did theirs. Even though they were employed by us, we grew to love them like they were part of our family.

There was a fine line, and it was hard to follow, especially for Giaci, who grew the most attached to his therapists. It was different from the relationship I had with my students; I was more disconnected from my class. I didn't see their homes or their personal lives, just their homework and school selves. Once someone stepped into your home, they were part of it.

THIRTY-SEVEN

An Unconventional Route

Over the next few years, I learned to adjust to our way of living. My ability to cope improved, especially as I saw Giaci master more and more skills. It was also a relief to see the girls and John adapting well to a constant stream of new therapists flowing in and out of our home. There had been so many changes in the early years, and we welcomed this period of steady growth. John and I were even able to give more attention to the girls' schooling and extracurricular activities and found more time for one another. No one was left out; no one was alone anymore.

We were chugging along comfortably until a new challenge presented itself: Giaci going to high school.

It had been a while since we last dreaded a school meeting, but this Individual Placement Review Committee meeting was important, and I was not looking forward to it. In it, we would discuss which high school Giaci would be attending in the fall.

For two years, we had visited potential high schools, asked questions and made requests in the hope that changes would be implemented by the time our son was ready to attend.

Despite all the time we spent visiting different locations, John and I still weren't satisfied. Not one classroom had met our son's needs or our expectations. We didn't see the level of behavioural methodologies being implemented that we were accustomed to and that Giaci needed to acquire necessary life and job skills.

Over the years, I'd learned that each skill Giaci acquired had to be based on his cognitive ability and needed to have a purpose in his life. Driving, unfortunately, was too complex of a skill with too many steps. Therefore, there was no need to teach him how to drive; functional skills were the most important. For example, we taught him how to use a washing machine to launder his clothes. Once again, the many steps involved in washing clothes were broken down for Giaci, and he learned them one at a time.

None of the schools offered anything comparable, and we had no idea where this meeting would go.

As we walked toward Giaci's school, Shoreline Elementary, for our meeting, one thing did feel different from past meetings like this: When Giaci was younger, I tended to shut myself down and not face the reality we were living with. Now I was armed with knowledge of autism and a solid understanding of what was best for Giaci and his future.

John and I met in the school parking lot as we had many times before; I was coming from home, and he was coming from work. We walked into the one-storey school building through the front entrance and made our way to the school office. There was a musty smell in the hallway that seemed all too familiar.

Having Giaci at this school for the past few years had been a fantastic experience for him and for us. Even though the other students also had high needs, the time and attention he received were far greater than what he would get if he had been in a mainstream classroom.

His classroom teacher was trained in applied behaviour analysis, and she had worked in a specialized clinical setting prior to becoming a teacher. She knew exactly how to teach Giaci, and she set him up for success. She shared her knowledge base with the support staff and her fellow teachers, and it grew from there, which positively affected Giaci's growth.

One important achievement was putting an end to his running-away behaviour. His teacher was intense in implementing and reinforcing appropriate behaviours, which ultimately stopped his impulsive need to dart off and run away. The collaboration between his home IBI team and the school programming solidified Giaci's skill retention.

This meeting was like many others, with John and I on one side of the table, outnumbered by those on the other side: the principal, classroom teacher, support staff, learning support teacher, and special education co-ordinator. It was hard not to replay the many times we'd been in this position before.

When the staff recommended a high school that we were *not* interested in, John and I looked at each other in disbelief. We wanted a high school that could teach him vocational skills, something that would allow him to work with his hands, perhaps custodial skills or a trade. We also wanted him to be taught personal life skills, like doing laundry or cooking his own food.

Now we were in a position to have to put our foot down and make the right decision for Giaci. With our combined strength, we turned down their proposal and excused ourselves from the table.

"Thank you for your time, but we will not be accepting your recommendation, and we will make other arrangements," John said with a calm and professional tone, and then we got up and walked out the door. The school officials were surprised to see us get up and leave like that. Their mouths dropped; they didn't know what else to say. Once upon a time we would have sat through the agony of them telling us why Giaci was suited for a particular space, but by now we knew what Giaci needed.

No, Giaci wouldn't be attending high school, and a part of me felt awful about him missing out on that pivotal teenage experience. But Giaci didn't understand any of that, and he didn't care because he didn't know what he was or wasn't missing. In time I realized that this alternative learning would benefit him more than any high school could. Giaci could do repetitive skills like wiping tables, refilling shelves, vacuuming, dusting. Once he learned a skill, he mastered it and he would puff up his chest with pride in accomplishing tasks. All his learning needs would be met by our staff, and he would have the opportunity to build social relationships with the staff at his work placements. We'd even incorporate social events into his schedule so we'd be sure he wasn't missing out on anything.

"We're going to do what we've always done: work it out," John said to me as we walked out. We would figure out a course of action that would be best for Giaci and our family.

After consulting with Dr. Barrera, our son's psychologist and also a board-certified behaviour analyst, we devised a unique plan for Giaci.

We were going to set up our own program to incorporate specialized academics, life skills, and job-skill training specifically made for Giaci. These were all functional skills that we felt were necessary for him to be an active part of the community as he grew into adulthood. This meant that Giaci would not be attending high school. Instead, we began transforming an area of our home into a classroom and scoping out locations in the community that would help Giaci generalize the skills he would learn in class.

Despite feeling like my blood was pounding in my head, I was ready to implement this unconventional and unique education. I was afraid of the unknown again but felt encouraged by the behaviour team we had assembled at home.

To make this work, I had to hire more staff who would be directed by the senior therapist and Dr. Barrera. It meant more work for me in overseeing the schedule, managing the payroll, and directing the teaching. But I knew that it was the best choice for all of us, especially Giaci.

John thought to use his community connections to help Giaci. "I'm going to call a few people in job-placement settings to see if Giaci can go there regularly," he said. John had this incredible way of helping me adjust to quick changes. His endless certainty was starting to rub off on me, and for once I was confident in our decision, too.

It was an unconventional route, but it felt right. We believed that we had a good grasp on Giaci's future, and we knew we had his best interests at heart.

THIRTY-EIGHT

A Happy-Go-Lucky Young Man

We started Giaci's work placements the summer before he turned fifteen. We had decided to teach him custodial skills, which he would be able to apply in actual job placements. These skills best suited his abilities, needs and physical strengths. Also, because he was a visual learner, it was easier to teach these skills through imitation.

With Giaci's team, we ironed out the details. We visited the offices in the municipal building, taking pictures of spaces so that Giaci could become familiar with them, speaking to the staff, and preparing for his daily arrival. The building supervisor, Sebastian, was supportive, and he took the initiative to make sure that his staff were aware of our objectives and Giaci's abilities. Sebastian was a man who took pride in his role, and he wanted to help Giaci succeed.

No amount of planning could have eased my nerves on Giaci's first official workday. We got him ready to leave the house, and he looked so grown up dressed in his full uniform. His therapists, Silena and Jaclyn, drove him to the office while I followed behind in my own car; I couldn't release my hold just yet. It was the overprotective mother in me that still had a hard time fully releasing him. I just wanted to make sure he had a good first day, to ease my mind.

It felt like his first day of kindergarten all over again. I'd held his hand so tight that day, fearing he'd run off. My hands trembled as I passed his hand over to his teacher's. I wasn't sure she would know how to keep him away from danger the way I did.

The difference today was that Giaci wasn't darting off. We'd all planned for this moment. Giaci had more skills under his belt than ever, and I had the ability to communicate both his and my needs. We were both ready to let go now.

Walking through the doors of the municipal building, Giaci was immediately greeted by everyone he encountered.

"Good morning, Giaci!" echoed through the corridors. A choir of supporters was what had been missing from our lives all along.

Giaci, recognizing that he was being spoken to, would answer with a stiff smile. He wasn't comfortable in the environment yet.

As Giaci and his therapists approached the elevator, I recognized his facial expression: it was a familiar look of apprehension. Giaci stood frozen, eyes widening with the opening elevator doors. He checked out the inside of the machine. He watched the patrons exit the elevator. He still stood motionless. I tried to keep my heart rate low so Giaci wouldn't notice the stress I felt deep in my bones.

"You can do it, buddy! You can do it!" I whispered under my breath.

Sebastian motioned with his hand, guiding Giaci to enter the elevator, and said, "After you, Mr. Giaci."

I held my breath as I watched from behind. Giaci scanned the elevator one more time and stutter-stepped forward as he looked over at Sebastian.

"Nice job, buddy!" I said instinctively, and Jaclyn laughed as the doors closed.

After that, the rest of Giaci's day was smooth and spectacular. Every skill he needed on-site was modelled, and he imitated it with precision. The fulfillment that came with accomplishing his duties brightened his face as he was praised not only by Silena and Jaclyn, but also by everyone he encountered. It was a community approach; we were all working as a collective to raise this young man.

As Giaci became more confident in his work, we expanded his duties to multiple locations, which also increased his skill set. At one building, he would deliver the newspaper to every office department. Each delivery increased his social interactions. We worked on social scripts so that he could have sentences practised and perfected to interact with co-workers.

"Good morning. How are you?" Giaci greeted the office administrator.

"I'm fine! How are you?" Emily answered, using the scripted responses.

Giaci's therapist Jaclyn had given Emily a few sentences to say that would prompt him to answer her in return. It may have seemed robotic and unnatural at first, but before long, the two became great pals, and they naturally had short, simple conversations. Emily even confided that talking to Giaci was the best part of her day. She was participating in his success and, just like the rest of the office, felt proud to watch his growth.

Years earlier, all I had wanted was for Giaci to be able to have a conversation with me. Now my wish was coming true. Not only could he have brief conversations with me, but he was also able to converse with others who enjoyed his presence and rejoiced in his accomplishments.

When he would come home, I'd ask him about his day.

"How was work today?"

"It was good, Mommy," he answered.

"What did you do?" I asked.

"I delivered the newspaper to the offices and cleaned the cafeteria," he said.

So many people commented on how much Giaci impressed them every day. It was more than I could ever have dreamed of for him.

In these moments, it was clear to me how much our society had evolved. In 2009, the province of Ontario had finally closed the doors of its last remaining institution-based facility, a place where those with autism and other intellectual disabilities were once hidden away from the community. Now, in 2010, my son was not only welcomed in the workplace but also loved as the happy-go-lucky, innocent young man he had become.

Our unique plan for our son was working. Not only was he progressing, but he was also positively affecting those around him. I relished this result of our decision to take the most unconventional route in Giaci's education. Now I could pull back and not hover over him and his therapists. I could focus on myself and my well-being.

I sometimes found myself thinking about Janice and Timothy, and I wondered how they were doing. I hadn't been able to reach Janice on the phone in some time as her number had been disconnected. I knew that she would have been happy to hear about Giaci's work success.

Eventually we added another work location to his schedule, and it quickly became his favourite place of all: the local nature centre. Giaci had always loved the outdoors, whether he was walking, running, swimming or just sitting under a tree. Nature had a calming effect on his demeanour and existence; it was his serene place. For this job, he fed the birds and walked the scenic nature trails, picking up the garbage that marred the picturesque view.

The picture-perfect scenery mirrored the beautiful life we had created for our son, a life I never could have envisioned when he was just a toddler: one with fresh air and meaning that would continue through adulthood.

THIRTY-NINE

Two Different Paths

Over the years, a persistent message had echoed within me: it was imperative for parents to learn behavioural strategies to achieve the best possible outcome for their children. Parents are with their child for the majority of the day, so it makes sense that these key players are the ones who need to be educated for the best results.

For so many years, I'd been told that getting involved with the autism community was crucial for Giaci's well-being—and my own—and now it was finally sinking in. This community and the connections we'd made through it had made the difference. Even though my life was still so busy with workshops, conferences, university classes and private coaching sessions, I knew involvement and engagement were essential. Being active in the autism community provided opportunities for research and fellowship, and allowed me to be a guest speaker, to raise funds and to make connections with professionals in the field that would improve Giaci's quality of life.

One year after Giaci started working, a professor from the University of Windsor called me and encouraged me to apply to teach part-time in the Autism and Behavioural Science graduate program at the college. I was still working as a full-time educator in the elementary school system, so adding this to my workload would be difficult, but the opportunity was meaningful for me and I knew it would be rewarding work. I applied and was accepted within a week.

As soon as the position started, I felt invigorated. I was able to share my knowledge while also providing a personal perspective as a parent. My role as a professor in the program was to monitor students in field placements, and I was helping educate professionals who would one day be working in the autism field. It didn't take long for me to learn how to balance all my duties, and my busy schedule made the years pass quickly.

One particular day started like any other: I was scheduled to meet with my college students at a community home location. It looked just like all the other homes on the block, but the inside was very different. As I stepped inside, I greeted the staff with a smile. I then met with my students in a private area tucked away in the back of the house.

We discussed their school assignments and schedules. The three clients in the home were on the autism spectrum, all with different ability levels. My students gave me a brief synopsis of each of them, with only their first names.

As we talked, they informed me that one of the three had severe behaviours and had been a challenge for the staff. Specialized staff had come in to implement behavioural techniques daily to address the aggression that erupted from this nonverbal young man. They were consulting with his psychiatrist to adjust his meds, hoping to calm his aggression. It took a multidisciplinary team approach with various clinicians to ensure that his needs were being addressed. His treatment was ongoing and ever changing.

My students were not assigned to work closely with him because of his extremely aggressive behaviours, but they were still involved in the team discussions on his care and behaviour intervention.

My students' heads bowed as they told me that the staff had been forced to confine this young man in an empty, locked room, as he could harm not only the staff but also himself.

They called this room the "calming room," but there was nothing calm about it. It was locked, and the only window in it was a peephole.

When I looked inside, I couldn't see the young man very well, but I could hear a loud, repetitive thumping sound.

"The staff tried to let him out yesterday," my student Sama informed me. She let her head hang. "It didn't go great. He had to be restrained and put back in the room." She blinked back tears. "I feel awful for him and his family. It's so upsetting." She blew her cheeks out with a thin breath. She then told me his parents had relinquished guardianship. The father had passed away, and the mother had been diagnosed with cancer and was unable to care for her son any longer.

"It's probably better that he doesn't understand what's happening," she said, trying to justify the terrible situation for this family.

My students and I continued our conferencing, focusing on the work that was being done. We skimmed over the visual schedules and other materials that were being used to help the clients in the home. As I glanced over their work, I noticed the aggressive young man's full name. The pictures then caught my eye.

Timothy.

Janice.

My eyes fogged up. The face in the photo wasn't the same face as the little boy who had been carried in his mother's loving arms when we went to see Dr. Krone more than ten years ago now. In this photo, he had a military buzzcut and a blank, expressionless face.

I started tipping over dizzily, unable to professionally process this situation. My students stared at me, wondering what I was mumbling. All I could say over and over again was "How?"

How did this happen?

How did Timothy get here?

Janice and I had started out together on the same path. *How had our paths diverged so sharply?*

All I could think of was her face. She had stunning, incredible features. They were more than enough to make her fascinating looking, not just attractive. Those same features were on the boy in the locked room. He too had mesmerizing ocean-blue eyes that compelled you to stare into them. My motherly instinct burned, producing a flaming desire to rip open the door and wrap my arms around Timothy with all the loving force a thousand mothers would possess.

My students finally broke through my distressed reaction.

"Are you all right, Rita? Is something wrong?" Sama asked. When I didn't respond, she asked again.

When I could finally speak, my voice glitched as if I were internally malfunctioning.

"Uh, yes…I'm okay…thanks. I know this boy." I regained enough composure to excuse myself and make my way to the door, completely forgetting for a moment why I was there to begin with.

I sprinted to my car, panting all the way. I tried to take in the reality of how different my son's life was from Timothy's. I still couldn't process that this was Janice's son's fate. We'd had the same dreams. We'd shared goals for our boys. I began sobbing. Janice and I hadn't spoken in years, but I could never have imagined the grossly different path she had been forced to take.

All I could think of was how hopeful we had been back then, when the boys were young. We were so driven to give our sons the absolute best outcome possible. Back then, we'd both wished for a crystal ball to look into the future and learn what was in store for our boys.

Neither of us could have imagined it would end like this, with Timothy locked in a room, without any stimulatory objects. It was a life of solitary confinement.

I wanted to call Janice that very moment, but the thought of her illness stopped me. So I called her cousin Hope.

"Hello, Hope, this is Rita."

"Hello, Rita." Her voice was subdued.

"How is Janice?" I asked.

"Not good—she isn't speaking and doesn't have much longer."

My heart ached for them.

"I'm so sorry. Please whisper a message to her from me. I want her to know that she was an incredible mother and she inspired me to never give up. Tell her I will keep a watchful eye on Timothy. We were on this journey together, and I won't ever forget that. I won't ever forget her."

Hope agreed to pass on my message, and we agreed to keep in touch for Timothy's sake. Even though I was devastated for Janice and Timothy, I was selfishly relieved that it wasn't *my* son in that room, locked away from all humanity. In my mind I kept repeating *There but for the grace of God go I*.

For years, John and I had worked so hard to keep our son constantly stimulated. We threw ourselves into behavioural intervention and consistent nutritional and naturopathic protocols. There were so many times when I wondered if what we were doing was enough or if it was all worth it.

The reality was that, no, Giaci wasn't "cured" or "recovered" from autism the way Janice and I had once hoped. All I knew was that my son, my Giaci, had autism for life, but that didn't mean he was suffering. I'd had to learn to let go of my own suffering to see that Giaci was happy. He was the happiest guy I knew, and we were all better for knowing and loving him.

Even though this wasn't how I had imagined my life, it was my uniquely perfect story. There was no magic, just a "doing the best we can" sort of life that required hard work every day.

The road we travelled, although rocky and unpleasant at times, wasn't pointless. Every day had precious gifts to be thankful for, and every day had purpose.

Giaci was that purpose.

FORTY

The Fullness of Life

I arrived home that day still lost in my thoughts, picturing Timothy on the other side of the door.

For years, I had envisioned and personified autism as a destructive force, one that had changed my family's life for the worse. But in reality, I just couldn't accept that the true beastly traits lay within *me*. I always focused on the negative and worried about things I couldn't control or change. I stressed about what others would think when it should never have mattered to me. I wasn't allowing myself to live; instead, I was wrapping myself in anger, denial and ego.

Within my cloak, I was accompanied by loud sabotaging voices telling me how I had failed my son, my family and myself. I couldn't shake the guilt that I couldn't cure Giaci of autism and that, because of me, our lives would never be perfect. For so long, the voices in my head told me that I was unworthy of a happy life. But as time passed and I became stronger, those voices got softer.

Only when I was able to push my ego aside could a powerhouse mother emerge. Only then could the astute soul within me surface and determine what was actually important in life. Only then could I make choices as a changed person, a new self, a new woman.

This journey with autism was as much my journey as it was my son's. We travelled it together as a family.

When John came home from work that day, I had to tell him about what happened. He had barely made it through the door before

I started detailing my encounter with Timothy and how different our lives could have been.

"I know, Rita. It's hard to imagine," he said, shaking his head in disbelief.

I hugged him close, grateful for my partner in parenting. "Even when you do everything right as a parent, things can still go wrong and not according to plan."

John nodded against the top of my head as I explained my epiphany.

"There isn't a formula to follow. No two stories are alike. We only know what we have gone through and how it has affected our family. We just need to enjoy every minute of it," I continued.

It was an awakening, an activation of a new self and a changed ego. A rush of self-compassion followed. I truly realized that I had to release my unhealthy attachment to what I had imagined for our lives. When I did so, peace settled in me. I realized that I had been blocking us from achieving my ultimate goal from the beginning: an enriched life, full of family and love…all of which had been right in front of me all along.

Only we mattered. Everything else ebbed and flowed, like the cyclical government autism programs. They shifted depending on who was in political power.

In 2019, things changed again. Since Giaci was now considered an adult, he wasn't affected by the government's decisions for ABA. The government in power erased years of advocating, years of fighting, and all our wins. They changed the way the funding was delivered to families and privatized the services. I was angry, but this was a fight for other parents now.

In 2020, when the COVID pandemic hit, we got the chance to slow down and reflect on our lives and all that had happened.

Lauren, who was living in Toronto to finish her studies to become a naturopathic doctor, came home. Carolina had almost finished her business degree, and Maria, who had followed in my footsteps to become a teacher, had just a year left before graduation.

All together again, we sat in the kitchen one night. The girls doted over their brother, as usual. Giaci was twenty-four years old now and all smiles, eating a big bag of chips without a care in the world. He was the centre of our family, and his joy in life was contagious.

John and I loved watching the raindrops fall, so we went out to the covered back porch and sat together to enjoy the nature sounds. The melodic pitter-patter of the rain hitting the roof shingles allowed us to relax. The earthy, citrusy smell of the geraniums cleared our minds.

In that moment, I thought about the many lessons we had learned throughout our journey. The one that stood out the most was that we hadn't moved on from autism: we had moved forward *with* autism. My determination to rid Giaci of this disability had been replaced by embracing who he was and how this had moulded us. My eyes had never been more open to the beauty of every little experience.

Giaci showed us how to enjoy the simplicity of life. Happiness for him was genuine and easy: a bag of chips, a big salad bowl or a Disney video would put him over the moon. There is a lot to be said about living this simply.

With the guidance of his therapists, Giaci continued to affect many people daily in our community. Even though we were still unable to have complex conversations with him, the life skills he had learned allowed him to be productive in our world while staying true to his own. Giaci demonstrated every single day what hard work was all about.

As much as I had wanted a life without autism, the reality was that autism would always be present in everything we did. It was present in the work I did, in the sculpting of the amazing women our girls had become, in John's vulnerability as a father, and in the precious person we all had in common: Giaci.

Giaci taught us that we needed to look within ourselves to understand our existence. He taught us to take each day one minute at a time, to not look forward or look back, and to cherish every moment.

After the rain stopped, the wind picked up, rattling the metal wind chimes and making a melodic clatter. John and I remained sitting on our patio chairs.

"You know, once the girls get married and leave, it's just me, you, and King Giaci," John mused with a satisfied smile.

"You got that right, honey. It's an Italian mother's dream to have her son living with her forever," I said.

Acknowledgements

In 2020, the twins, Carolina and Maria, created a TikTok account and posted a video of them doing an art activity with their brother. When that video went viral, Carolina continued to create videos because followers were asking for "more Giaci." The more the girls posted, the more Giaci was viewed and the more popular he became. This is not to say we gained fame, rather a lot of attention from all over the world. The videos were not only playful but also educational. Social media allowed us to share stories, to educate, to connect with parents, grandparents, professionals in the field and other autistics. It was all-encompassing. Followers were inquiring about our family's journey and how we got to adulthood with Giaci.

Giaci and Me is relevant today because it helps people understand what families with an autistic child experience. My hope is that by reading this book, students and professionals will find new ways to better serve the autistic community, gain a greater understanding of the cultural influences neurodivergent people both offer and are impacted by, and find empathy for their situations.

In telling our family's story, I have endeavoured to educate readers about cultural norms, controversies, different perspectives, language, ableism, neurodiversity and behavioural intervention. It depicts a mother's deep affection and unwavering strength to pursue acceptance rather than anger, shame and resentment. It is a story of reshaping viewpoints despite uncovering my flaws to create a foundation of growth and change. Through the ups and downs, I never lose sight of who I was and how I came to be the woman I am today.

While there is still a lot of life to live, I can truthfully say that I have been changed for the better because of my son's autism diagnosis. I have gained a sense of self-worth permeated by this journey gifted to me as a mother of an autistic child, and I look forward to whatever new lessons I learn next.

To express my deep gratitude for support on this journey, I would like to acknowledge my husband John, and my daughters, Lauren, Carolina and Maria, for their constant support, unity, love, understanding and patience.

Very special thanks also to family and friends, therapists who have come and gone over the years, professionals in the field, and other parents of autistic children that I have had the privilege to walk alongside. Thanks to my publisher Genevieve Loughlin, editorial director Mo Duffy Cobb, managing editor Renée Layberry, designer Jordan Beaulieu, and sensitivity reader Shannon Bruyneel, for their keen sense of professionalism and attention to detail. And to Alley Biniarz for the constant encouragement I needed to finish my book

Above all, I'd like to thank my son, Giaci, the one who grounds me and is the centre of our family. He has been my most tenacious teacher in life, guiding me on how to fully accept others for who and how they are, showing me what unconditional love is, enriching my own personal growth and self-awareness. He has opened my eyes to see the beauty in celebrating all things great and small and has shown me that we continue to learn every day no matter what age we are. He is sunshine and has given me the light I needed when I could only see darkness.

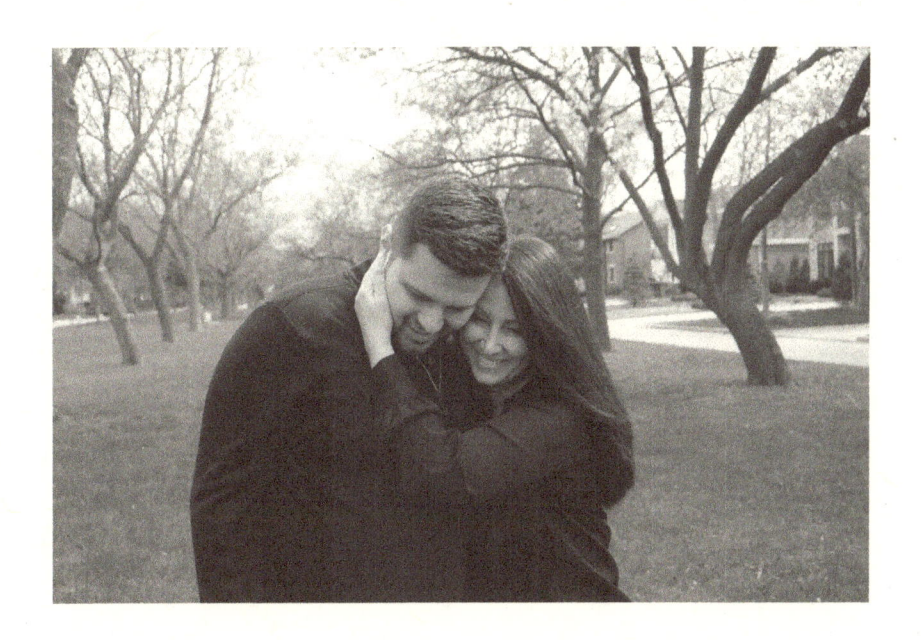

RITA MICELI

A life-long educator and a long-time advocate for autism awareness, Rita Miceli is a contributor in the international bestselling book *Ambitious Women Rise: The Amazing Stories of Women Overcoming Obstacles and Creating the Life of Their Dreams*. As an educator for over three decades, Miceli teaches in the Autism and Behavioural Science Graduate Program at St. Clair College. She and her family have been featured in *The Drive Magazine*, on CTV news and on CBC National News. Rita is the past president of Autism Ontario (Windsor/Essex Chapter) and has published works on multiple platforms related to the topics of special needs and autism, including *A Call to Action* (Autism Matters) and *Words that Connect Us* (Canadian Authors Association). She won the Best New Canadian Manuscript award from the Word Guild for her manuscript entitled *Giaci and Me: Life Lessons on Raising an Autistic Child*. Rita lives in Windsor, Ontario, with her high school sweetheart, John, and is the proud mother of three daughters and an autistic son.